Why Not Me?

Pamalla Stockho

Maggie Garfield, editor
Jane Boynton, cover artist

Although this is a work of non-fiction, all patient names have been changed. Some of the patient encounters are composites of similar cases. Patients are representative of nearly a quarter of a century of nursing practice. Not all visits portrayed were specific to the Family Medical Center. Any resemblance to individuals either living or dead, outside of those listed on the dedication and acknowledgment pages, is purely coincidental.

National Library of Canada Cataloguing in Publication Data

Stockho, Pamalla, 1953-
    Why not me?

ISBN 1-55369-113-X

    1. Stockho, Pamalla, 1953- —History. 2. Breast—Cancer—Patients—United States—Biography. I. Title.

RC280.B8S76 2002   362.1'9699449'0092   C2001-904020-2

TRAFFORD

This book was published *on-demand* in cooperation with Trafford Publishing.
On-demand publishing is a unique process and service of making a book available for retail sale to the public taking advantage of on-demand manufacturing and Internet marketing.
On-demand publishing includes promotions, retail sales, manufacturing, order fulfilment, accounting and collecting royalties on behalf of the author.

Suite 6E, 2333 Government St., Victoria, B.C. V8T 4P4, CANADA
Phone   250-383-6864   Toll-free   1-888-232-4444 (Canada & US)
Fax   250-383-6804   E-mail   sales@trafford.com
Web site   www.trafford.com   TRAFFORD PUBLISHING IS A DIVISION OF TRAFFORD HOLDINGS LTD.
Trafford Catalogue #01-0515   www.trafford.com/robots/01-0515.html

10   9   8   7   6   5   4

Dedicated, with love, to

Dan Lansing, who won his battle with cancer;

Cathy Comstock, who soars with angels;

and Michael Littwin, whose brain tumor, thankfully,

proved to be benign.

Acknowledgments

I will be eternally grateful for the patience and understanding shown me during the interminably long period of editing, editing, and more editing shown me by my husband, *Bill*, and my three children: *Heather*, *Jonathan*, and *Robert*. They lovingly put up with my splashing their names and lives across these pages.

I am very thankful to all the colleagues, friends, and family who graciously lent their names and support for my book: Eileen and Jim Abbott; Tricia Anson; Norman Aarestad, M.D.; Gloria Bachelder, M.D.; Linda and David Bailey; Jennifer Bowers, M.A.; Nadine Farquhar; Carol Gleeson; Janis Green; Debra Gruich, R.N.; Patty Harper, R.N.; Chris Hibbard, Ph.D.; H. David Hibbard, M.D.; Kari Hyde; Charles Jones, M.D.; Anne Marie and James Kennedy; Barb Lansing, R.N.; Cindy and Michael Littwin; Dan Martin, R.N.; Eilish McCafferty; Lisa McCoy; Lee McNeely, M.D.; Lou Ann Perko, R.N.; Sharon Pittenger, M.D.; Krystal Reider, M.A.; Gail Reinke, R.N.; James Richard, M.D.; Joyce Ross, R.N.; Mark Sitarik, M.D.; Debbie Smith, Radiation Therapist; Tina Suleski, R.N.; Judy Walton, F.N.P.; Connie Wilson, R.N.; and, of course, Mom and Dad.

WHY NOT ME?

Preface

I am a breast cancer survivor, but I haven't just survived. I embrace fun and passion, challenging myself to envision a better version of the woman I've become. The patients I treat, the family I adore, and the friends in whom I rejoice enhance each day and every treasured memory.

I will not dispute the beliefs of those who claim cancer did not change them, but subtle modifications in my attitude and expectations built gradually to dramatically redefine the person I was. I laugh often, listen more intently, speak less, and take the time—I swore I never had—to pursue loves I have nurtured since my treatments ended: tackling a new language, learning to play musical instruments, sharing jokes until my face hurts from smiling, embracing the Irish culture, and writing. The writing, begun during my ordeal to help me cope with being slapped in the face with my mortality, has lifted my spirit and driven me to excel.

Indulgent friends find my love of a people so different from my own an enigma. However, while I battled cancer, I absorbed eight hundred years of Irish struggling to preserve life and culture. The tenacity of the Irish people spoke volumes to me in my despair. The love remains, helped in generous measure by dear Irish friends like Anne Marie and James Kennedy (County Galway, Republic of Ireland), and Eileen and Jim Abbott (County Antrim, Northern Ireland). I will let the psychologists make what they will of my devotion.

I rejoice in small daily accomplishments instead of hoping for ecstasy in the nebulous future. Of course, I still have bad days—when I'm grumpy, don't want to work, don't want to pick up the house—but those days are relatively few and friends like Anne Marie slap the self-pity out of me with comments like (Irish accent here): "Are you going to stand around all night with that face on you?"

My life enriches with each person I meet. I liberally infuse my clinical practice with heavy doses of patience and compassion, but I'm not a nauseatingly bubbly, sappy, proselytizing sprite who needs a reality check or kick in the *arse*. I enjoy spirited dialogue, encourage divergent views, and thrive on humor.

I am not glad I had cancer, but life has been spectacular since the battle. If I die an old woman, I'll know I beat the disease; if not, I'll have made my peace with most of my faults, despite my perpetual guilt for imagined sins ingrained in parochial school.

Paradoxically, I talk to God more often and follow the tenets of my religion less. He is never far from my thoughts, although I'm sure He understands I am in no hurry to shake His hand. He is more than symbols of faith or buildings of worship to me, and I enjoy greeting Him each day as I absorb myself in the beauty of the mountains near my home or in the smile of a child who has survived examination by his nurse practitioner—me.

My story is not a sugarcoated fairy tale, for that is not how my life has been. It involves pain as well as happiness—both my patients' and mine. I have been privileged to care for many people during twenty-six years of nursing service, and in their own ways, they have cared for and nurtured me as well. I am a hard-working wife, mother, and nurse practitioner, who, like other women diagnosed with breast cancer, was forced to re-evaluate goals and priorities. I could not rely on fame, riches, or a body to die for to help me through my ordeal.

Speaking of fame, riches, and a body to die for, a patient of mine advanced the hypothesis that everyone chooses a body and pattern of life before birth. She believes God encourages choice based on lessons the soul requires for growth. I'm not sure I believe in reincarnation, with apologies to Shirley MacLaine, but if such a plan exists, I don't recall choosing to be a short, calorie-challenged woman with breast cancer. However, if I did select this life, I will just say, "Lord, whatever lessons I needed to learn, I have learned them. Honest! In my next life, please make me 5'10", beautiful, and rich. And I'd appreciate keeping the intelligence I've developed in this life as well. Amen."

Cancer does not end life for most of us these days. The sun continues to rise and set, and I've learned to cherish the moment. I hope this book brings a bit of knowledge and comfort to those facing similar trials. Perhaps a smile or two will ease the journey.

Chapter 1 - December 14th, 1998

My tranquil mood evaporated abruptly Monday morning when an elderly woman, who I will charitably call eighty-something, sailed through a red light and stopped within an inch of plowing into my Saturn. The woman's saucer-sized eyes peeking over the steering wheel blinked rapidly and blankly behind coke-bottle-thick eyeglasses. She finally focused on me and stared for a second before she backed up and drove off, leaving me shaking in the intersection. A horn honked and startled me into movement. I made it to work on autopilot.

I walked past the Louisville Family Medical Center's front desk and stared at the patient care providers' schedules that were tacked to the bulletin board. Among four providers, there were only six available patient appointments for the entire day. I considered all the patients who would call for same day appointments and sighed. Mondays generally proved frustrating for both staff and patients.

Our deteriorating medical building was built nearly fifteen years ago, when Dr. David Hibbard started his practice. If a tornado had ripped through it, taking every ancient exam table and broken gooseneck lamp, I would have praised heaven. It was embarrassing escorting patients to cramped, drab, examination rooms. The worn, gray carpet hadn't weathered the episodic bouts of vomit and blood that left unsightly stains, many of which successfully withstood frequent carpet cleanings. The faded wallpaper was curling, helped in part by young patients surreptitiously peeling the edges as they waited impatiently for their visits.

Those young patients were proof of the many Louisville families who evolved with our clinic. Due to the burgeoning patient population in booming Louisville, the building was bursting at its seams, but there was no room for expansion to accommodate desperately needed providers and staff.

I deposited my derriere into my padded desk chair and perused the stacks of patient charts waiting for my signature on prescription refills; laboratory, radiology, mammogram, and Pap reports; and dictated progress notes from specialists who'd seen my patients. I scanned notes clipped to charts by the phone nurse to ensure none required my immediate attention. As I pored over a mammogram report, a voice on the clinic's intercom clamored insistently.

"Pam Stockho, stat, Room 1! Stat, Room 1!"

Leaping to my feet too quickly, I slammed my left knee into the desk. I limped down the narrow hallway to examination Room 1 and ignored stares from co-workers well acquainted with my less than graceful ability to navigate the narrow hallways. Trying to distract my mind from my knee pain, I marveled that I'd been employed in the clinic as a family nurse practitioner for nearly four years. I married a U.S. naval officer, a submarine commander, and never lived in any city long enough to hold a job for more than three years—until he retired. For the first time in over twenty years of marriage, I felt settled. The thought was comforting, but my knee still hurt.

While I daydreamed about a promised larger, new clinic with state-of-the-art equipment, I tripped over a worn bit of carpeting. I uselessly shot my hand out, vainly clutching at the wall to keep from falling. I managed to further wrench my knee in the process. Righting myself, I smoothed out the wretched carpet. I cut through the nurse's station to save a few seconds, earning me dirty looks from bodies I accidentally goosed in my haste.

I avoided the slow ceiling leak one of the nurses had enterprisingly stemmed with a duct-taped disposable diaper. It hung ominously low following two weeks of unseasonable thunderstorms. The staff had placed bets on which nurse or provider would be the recipient of the impending deluge. With my luck, or lack thereof, I probably faced a major drenching. In fact, bets were running four to one in my favor of winning the dubious honor.

I burst into Room 1. Barb, one of the clinic's stellar R.N.s, stood at the head of the exam table holding an oxygen mask over the face of a very frightened woman. That assumption came from noting the patient's wildly dilated eyes, both of which fixated on me the instant I crossed the threshold. Ashen-faced, with areas of red, raised splotches and hives, the fifty-two year old woman sat bolt upright, breathing rapidly. She grasped ineffectively at the oxygen mask.

Oh, oh! I thought. The differential diagnosis list that skipped through my mind was short and anaphylaxis—a severe allergic reaction—topped it. Without rapid intervention, she could stop breathing. My chest tightened and my heart pounded wildly. Just because I had to look calm didn't mean I always felt that way.

Barb provided a synopsis of the situation. "Pam, Mrs. Jenkins walked into the clinic five minutes ago. Dr. Richard ordered an antibiotic, cephalexin, on Saturday morning for her eye infection. Itching began last night. After this morning's dose, she experienced shortness of breath and broke out in hives. Instead of going to the emergency room, she came here."

Barb rolled her eyes, but there was no sense telling the patient she'd made a serious error in judgment coming to the clinic instead of going to the ER five minutes away, or calling 911 when her respiratory distress escalated. Just like on television, our local emergency room dealt with almost any acute situation. Our small clinic wasn't set up to manage potentially life-threatening conditions. We handled basic emergencies, sure, but this situation was different. Mrs. Jenkins' problem was turning very nasty, very quickly.

Barb continued. "None of the doctors has arrived yet. Since you're on the scene, you were elected."

Why me? I thought; on the other hand, why not me?

Mrs. Jenkins' wild eyes darted from one nurse to another. Her respiratory rate increased. Beads of sweat saturated her forehead. I took a deep breath, managed a half-hearted smile, and walked to the exam table. I clasped the woman's clammy hand in mine.

"Mrs. Jenkins, I'm Pam Stockho, the nurse practitioner here. We're going to help you. Do you have any allergies to medicines?" I asked. Other than this one, I thought. She shook her head.

I looked at the nurses, each one capable in dealing with situations like these. How many times had I watched medical interns and residents new to the ER nervously beg help from nurses who'd seen years of crises?

Sounding like a drill sergeant, I barked orders for medications that would hopefully stop the drug reaction. Then I silently prayed. Please God, let that happen instead of the situation deteriorating further.

"Barb, give her 0.3cc of epinephrine subcutaneously." I turned to Lou Ann and Tina, both clinic R.N.s awaiting orders. "Lou Ann, start an IV of D5W to keep a vein open and give Benadryl 25 mg IV. Tina, call 911 for an ambulance and prod the first doctor who arrives in this direction."

I ordered a blood pressure reading and listened to Mrs. Jenkins' back with my stethoscope—wheezes everywhere. Her respiratory rate reached fifty. I lifted the back of the exam table so she could lean against it while maintaining the upright position that would ease her breathing.

"Mrs. Jenkins." I willed myself to speak calmly in spite of my increasing anxiety. My legs felt rubbery. The frightened woman stared blankly at the pictures of Dr. Richard's family gracing one wall. I took her face in my hands and looked directly into her eyes.

"Mrs. Jenkins. Try to slow your breathing down—you're hyperventilating because you're scared. Are you feeling dizzy?"

Mrs. Jenkins nodded warily. Her gray hair lay in damp ringlets on her forehead. I squeezed her hand gently.

"Do your fingertips and mouth feel tingly?" I asked.

The frightened woman nodded again.

"Ok." I asked Tina to check a pulse ox to determine how saturated her blood was with oxygen. I imagined it would approach 100% with the oxygen she was receiving by mask and her hyperventilation. I was right.

"Oxygen saturation is 100%, and her pulse is 108."

Quietly I said, "I'll remove the oxygen. Cup a hand over your face to re-breathe some of your own air. You'll feel less dizzy. Try to slow down your breathing. Trust me. I won't leave you." No, I thought, I can't leave. You're gripping my left hand like a piece of wood in a vice. Perhaps a nice X-ray to look for fractures would be appropriate after the crisis passes.

I ordered another blood pressure and continued chatting in hopes of pacifying her fear...and mine. Thankfully, Mrs. Jenkins was unaware of my rapidly beating heart. Nothing says, "Oh shit!" quicker than realizing your health care provider is on the verge of panic.

Had I been in a fully equipped emergency room, I would not have been panicking. But our emergency equipment consisted of a couple of pediatric-sized endotracheal tubes, a laryngoscope, EKG machine, oxygen, and a bottle of 1:1000 epinephrine. That was not exactly an inventory of emergency equipment that would instill warm fuzzies in anyone coping with a potentially life-threatening situation. Our clinic was not permitted to have a crash cart and emergency equipment, because it opened a whole can of worms regarding accreditation. As useless as it had been to maintain my Advanced Cardiac Life Support certification, I was reticent to drop it, and I cringed every time a crisis occurred. Thankfully, they were rare. Most patients knew to go to the ER in an emergency.

"Mrs. Jenkins, you've developed an allergy to your antibiotic. We're giving you medicines to stop the reaction." Please, God, make it so. "An ambulance will take you to the emergency room so you can be watched for a few hours. You may be admitted overnight."

Lou Ann wiped Mrs. Jenkins' forehead with a cool cloth. The patient's respiratory rate slowed, and her death grip on my hand lessened. Her arms and legs began to relax slightly. I listened to her back again and heard fewer wheezes. The meds were working, thank God!

"You're doing great!" I assured her.

"Pam, what have we got here?" Dr. Hibbard demanded, striding into the room a few minutes later. He pulled a stethoscope from his pants pocket. Dr. Hibbard, the clinic founder, embodied the oft-used phrase "aging gracefully". At sixty-one, the man looked at least ten years younger. His finely chiseled features were appreciated by many of the women seen in our clinic. As those thoughts crossed my mind, I could just hear the nurses say, "Oh don't tell him that! He's hard enough to live with as it is!"

"Dr. Hibbard, Mrs. Jenkins is a fifty-two year old woman who started cephalexin Saturday for peri-orbital cellulitis. She started itching last night. She broke out in hives and became short of breath after her dose of antibiotic this morning. Her last blood pressure was 104/60. It usually runs about 122/70. It's been ten minutes since her injection of epinephrine and five minutes since she received IV diphenhydramine, and her lungs are beginning to clear."

I turned to Tina. "Please repeat a blood pressure."

"It's 108/64, Pam."

"Ladies, it appears Dr. Hibbard won't have to intubate." I glanced at Mrs. Jenkins. I didn't explain my comment, but she would probably have been thrilled to learn we weren't going to stick a child-sized tube down her trachea to assist breathing.

"Terrific, Pam," Dr. Hibbard said. "I haven't intubated a patient in several years. The ambulance has arrived. You give report and I'll call the ER physician. I'll be in my office if you need me—my first patient was scheduled for a physical and hasn't shown up yet."

The rest of the morning proved to be typically Monday, with one patient disaster after another. None of us was spared. To accommodate the post-weekend demand, extra patients were worked into the already full provider schedules.

At lunchtime, Barb accosted me in the kitchen. "Pam, a new patient is at the front desk. He's had abdominal pain for four days. His wife phoned their insurance company Friday evening. They suggested he call his primary care physician before going to the emergency room, but he's only recently moved here and hasn't established care yet. He didn't know how to contact us over the weekend, so he waited until today. The doctors have already left the building—something about continuing education at Avista Hospital. I felt uncomfortable having him wait until after lunch."

"Bring him to Room 1, Barb." I certainly couldn't complain. Usually the docs got stuck working through lunch. I was generally able to stuff my face while I finished writing up patient charts from the morning.

I'd only half-listened to her comments. "What did his insurance company tell him, Barb?"

"They told his wife he would be responsible for the cost of an ER visit if it wasn't a true emergency. He doesn't have much money, so he waited until he could come in today. His wife left work at lunchtime to bring him over."

"Where's his pain?" I asked.

"Right lower quadrant."

"Want to bet he has a hot appendix? If he perforates after waiting all weekend to be seen, his insurance company will get an earful from me!"

I stopped at the Lilliputian-sized nurse's station to calm down. An unbelievable amount of paraphernalia was crammed into it, including one refrigerator for medications and another for blood requiring transit to labs throughout the city. A microscope allowed us to diagnose basic vaginal infections and sexually transmitted diseases (STDs). Nebulizer treatments to ease breathing were available. Supplies needed to draw blood and give immunizations were housed there.

The nurses organized paperwork and reference books in the nurse's station as well. They advised us when we needed pre-authorization to beg for necessary patient medications from insurance companies, whose lists of allowed drugs changed frequently, depending on cost and monetary incentives from drug companies.

Dealing with insurance companies frequently infuriated me, especially when they hired people with little medical knowledge. Those individuals occasionally made ludicrously inappropriate decisions regarding patients' medical conditions. Our doctors often questioned the point of having gone to medical school when "some bimbo with a high school diploma denies requisite care".

Until HMOs were held accountable for devastating medical decisions, the system would continue to put patients at unnecessary risk. Of course, not all insurance companies were guilty, but people often didn't discover their health care policy limitations until a crisis arose.

I certainly hoped a critical situation wasn't brewing in Room 1. Barb walked out of the room and handed me the patient's chart.

"His temperature is 103, Pam. He's writhing in pain."

I opened the door. A short, dark-skinned man squirmed on the exam table. He perspired profusely. A petite, dark-haired woman stood beside him, wringing her hands. Her eyes shot from me to the man.

"Mr. and Mrs. Kushal, I'm Pam Stockho, the clinic's nurse practitioner. Mr. Kushal, I would like to help alleviate your suffering as quickly as possible. How long have you had this pain?"

"My English not so good. My wife…"

"He's had pain on and off for four days," Mrs. Kushal told me. "It's been steady since last night."

"Has he thrown up?" I asked.

"No," the woman responded after conversing in Urdu with her husband. "But he wants to."

"Any fever before today?"

"No, I don't think so." I watched the woman's worried eyes scrutinize the room, which doubled as a procedure and examination room. It looked shabbier to me than usual. Mrs. Kushal stared at the pictures of Dr. Richard's family, much as Mrs. Jenkins had earlier.

Mr. Kushal moaned, snapping his wife's attention back to him. A look of despair crossed her face.

"Mrs. Kushal, has he had any chills?" The woman closed her eyes.

"Mrs. Kushal? Are you all right?"

"Yes. What is wrong with my husband?" Tears trickled down her face.

I responded gently. "I need to examine him and run some tests before I can answer with certainty. Just a few more questions, please."

"Are you a doctor?" The woman's lower lip trembled.

"No, ma'am. I chose to become a nurse practitioner because I love nursing. I have been a nurse for twenty-three years. Doctors go to medical school. I have a master's degree in nursing and twelve years of experience as a nurse practitioner."

"Do you and the doctors see different kinds of patients?"

"No, although I generally care for more patients with acute problems. If one of my patients requires admission, I review orders with the doctor on call. I promise to take good care of your husband."

She nodded.

I touched the woman's arm. I wanted to assure her of my competence, but felt we needed to focus on the problem at hand. "Let's return to your husband. Before my examination, I need to ask a few more questions. The answers will help me identify the cause of his pain."

By the end of the exam, it was fairly obvious this was a textbook case of appendicitis, although I could count on one hand the number of textbook cases I'd seen. Appendicitis frequently presented in diagnostically challenging ways. While a stat blood count was run, I called a surgeon. I would later learn that within two hours, Mr. Kushal was on an operating room table, having his inflamed appendix removed.

"Isn't it great when everything flows well like that?" I remarked to Sophia, the front desk wizard who managed patient flow. "I love it! Bring on the next patient." I paused. "Wait! Maybe I'll grab a quick bite first."

After inhaling my lunch and popping a Pepcid AC to ward off postprandial indigestion, a common affliction in our overworked clinic, I spent the next hour and a half on routine physicals and Paps. Patients in our clinic were usually scheduled at fifteen-minute intervals, with more time allotted for physical examinations and complex problems. Although fifteen minutes was enough time to deal with one or two concerns, patients frequently harbored hidden agendas, which they failed to convey to appointment clerks. Often those problems were mentioned to the provider in passing at the conclusion of a visit.

Some of those "Oh, by the ways..." couldn't be put off until another appointment time. When a patient casually mentioned he'd been "having a little chest pain when I play golf..." at the end of an appointment made for allergies, I couldn't ignore *that*, could I? Most patients accepted the occasional emergency with grace and understanding, but I always felt like a kid arriving late to school without a note from my mother when I apologized for my tardiness. Occasionally, the appointment clerks allotted too little time for a complex condition, but regardless of the reason, getting behind proved frustrating, and I'd be the first to admit I didn't always handle frustrations gracefully.

Paged from my office, where I was catching up on charts, I walked down the hall to Room 5 to see Mr. Anderson. His chief complaint was: "follow-up appointment from my emergency room visit".

I noticed the dour look on the patient's wife's face as soon as I entered the room. A pinched expression and raised eyebrow spoke volumes despite her silence. Her arms were crossed defiantly, and she glared at him from across the room. I sat at the desk beside Mr. Anderson, angling my chair so I could observe him easily. He glanced up at me and smiled shyly.

"What took you to the emergency room, Mr. Anderson?"

"I fell out of a tree," he said sheepishly.

"Tell her the whole truth," his wife spat out.

He sighed. "My wife plays bingo most Wednesdays down at the church. When she's gone, and when it's a full moon, I climb a tree in our back yard, carrying a six-pack of Bud. I climb up to this branch that's about thirty feet up, never had no problem before, and drink my beers." He gave his wife a furtive glance and scratched his head.

Thus encouraged, she said, "Go on. Tell her everything. Tell her how you sit up there and interfere with yourself. Go on."

My mind wandered back to parochial school and Sister telling us it was a sin to interfere with yourself. There'd been lots of giggling. I stifled that urge as I looked at Mr. Anderson. He glanced at me and smiled sheepishly. I was about to tell him to skip the details, when his wife piped up again.

"Go on. Tell her."

He coughed. "After I drink my beers, I howl at the moon for a while. Then I jack off. I don't cause nobody no problem, and the missus knows nothing about it."

"Ha!" His wife fixed him with a look that withered the man where he sat. "But the bingo game was cancelled, so I was walking under that damn tree to the house just as he was, you know, spraying the yard. Well, I got sprayed and screamed and this moron fell out of the tree onto his back. I was so pissed; I beat him with my purse the whole time we were in the ambulance. It's too bad he didn't bust something else coming out of that tree, 'cause he ain't going to be using that little part for a while—that's for damn sure."

I covered my mouth to stifle what might have been an embarrassing guffaw. Partially recovering my professionalism, I asked, "Where do you hurt, sir?"

"My shoulder blade mostly—and my hip."

I checked his skin for bruises before examining him. I poked and probed, finding a very tender right scapula. Movement at his shoulder shot waves of pain through his shoulder blade. I sent him for X-rays of his scapula. Pictures of his shoulder, hip, and ribs taken in the ER had shown no fractures.

Two of our nursing wonders, Lou Ann and Krystal, doubled as X-ray techs in our office, but our X-ray equipment would have been considered state-of-the-art only to Madame Curie. Beyond basic limb, chest, or abdominal films, we sent patients to the urgent care down the street.

While I waited for Mr. Anderson to return with his films, I grabbed Alex Turnbull's chart from the rack beside Room 7. I glanced at the chief complaint: "sports physical for football". Area coaches demanded the blessings of a health care provider before allowing their charges to be mangled, maimed, and lacerated. At least the exam should be straightforward, I thought. The afternoon was proving to be infinitely more pleasant than the morning had been.

My twelve-year-old patient sat on the exam table, flexing his biceps muscles. Dressed in a T-shirt of purple, black, and silver, emblazoned with the Rockies baseball team logo, I took a calculated risk in asking if he were a Rockies fan. Okay, so I'm not a great sports aficionado. I can't be good at everything.

"I'm a big Rockies fan, Mrs. Stockho. But I want to play football this year." Near the end of the exam, while I examined muscles and joints, I asked about any problems associated with them. Alex beamed with pride.

"What?" I demanded, knowing that a high school male is usually *that* proud only about something he does better than his pals. I was right. Alex routinely entertained his friends by dislocating his left shoulder at will. He proceeded to demonstrate, easily crunching and popping the head of the humerus back into place. His father, standing beside him, shuddered at the exhibition.

Alex grinned. "Sometimes it pops out all by itself. I was wondering something though, Mrs. Stockho."

"Yes?" I asked.

"Have you ever seen any of those *Lethal Weapon* movies with Mel Gibson?"

"I have."

"You know when his shoulder pops out of the joint and he bangs himself against walls and stuff to get it back in?"

Now it was my turn to shudder. "Uh huh."

"Well, that never works for me. You wanna see?"

"I'll pass, thanks. And I wouldn't advise it. Mr. Gibson's movies should come with a disclaimer—something like: 'Don't try this at home'. Popping your arm in and out of its socket is an interesting trick, and although the rest of your exam is normal, I can't sign your sports form. You need to see an orthopedic specialist. That's a bone doctor." He looked dejected. I felt sorry for him, but my primary professional objective had always been to avoid amplifying problems. Hippocrates said it best when he admonished medical practitioners to "do no harm".

After Alex, I saw a couple of ladies for their annual Pap exams and reviewed medications for patients with diabetes, high blood pressure, and congestive heart failure. Rounding out the afternoon was an embarrassed woman with a potato-sized geode in her vagina, placed there the evening before when she'd had one beer too many; a gentleman with a pus-filled abscess requiring incision and drainage; a five-year-old boy with a scalp laceration, who'd run into a table rather than around it; and a teenage boy with a wrist fracture sustained while snowboarding. I was definitely ready to call it a day when Barb grabbed me.

"Pam, I've a work-in for you. Guy can't breathe. He's in Room 5."

"Oh, man! I hope the day isn't going to end the way it started." I moved quickly to Room 5. "Did you get an oxygen saturation?" I knew she would have.

"Ninety-four percent," Barb responded.

"Okay."

The middle-aged man, Mr. Bennett, was breathing rapidly at about thirty-six breaths per minute.

"How long has this been going on?" I removed my stethoscope from around my neck.

"Since last night." He struggled to say the words before taking a breath, which precipitated coughing spasms. "Can't get my breath. Had a cold last two days. Thought I was getting better, but today worse."

"Any history of asthma or other respiratory illnesses other than an occasional cold?"

He shook his head.

"Do you smoke?" I considered the question rhetorical since his clothing reeked of cigarettes.

"Smoke two packs a day."

"Do you have any allergies to medicine?"

Again he shook his head.

"Are you taking any medications or herbs every day?"

"No."

I scanned his chart. "You had a chest X-ray two months ago when you had a physical."

He nodded.

After listening to his wheeze-filled lungs, and to his heart, which was beating regularly at ninety-two beats per minute, I stuck my head out the door. I requested a nebulizer treatment to open his air passages.

"I'll leave the door open in case you need anything, Mr. Bennett. This inhalation treatment will get medicine into your lungs to ease your breathing. It may make you shaky and dizzy. I'll return to listen to your lungs after your treatment. Barb will stay with you until you feel better, and I'll check on you frequently. The treatment lasts about ten minutes."

Surprisingly clear of wheezes after one treatment, I examined him for signs of illness. He had an upper respiratory infection, but it took a couple of minutes to convince him he needed an inhaler and not antibiotics for his virus. I demonstrated proper use of the inhaler and asked him to call if he had further problems.

After discharging Mr. Bennett, I made my way to my office and collapsed into a chair, saying to no one in particular, "Thank God this day is over! It sure was a Monday."

Chapter 2 - December 17th

The University of Colorado at Boulder boasted a beautiful campus. Nestled among the foothills of the Flatiron Mountains, one was afforded the illusion of a serene, pastoral setting, although the school was located in the picturesque town of Boulder.

The town was quaint. Centrally located, the Pearl Street Mall shops opened onto a bricked promenade, where street vendors and minstrels entertained daily, asking only a few coins for their efforts. Aging hippies held court amid hordes of pedestrians. Outdoor cafes, with their savory aromas, lured famished shoppers. Many emporiums offered the heterogeneous works of gifted local artisans. Elsewhere in town, herbal shops and health food stores abounded, appeasing the diverse idiosyncrasies of inhabitants and transients.

Boulder residents heartily espoused the university. At games, there were nearly as many gaily-clad alumnae as there were students sporting the black and gold colors of the Colorado Buffaloes football team.

The school buildings at the University of Colorado at Boulder, otherwise known as CU Boulder, were constructed of rust and sand-colored stone, giving the campus the appearance it naturally evolved from the surrounding environment. Well, maybe not the whole campus. The dorms known as the Quad, four older buildings housing engineering students, looked more like rejected WWII Army billets than homes away from home.

My son, Jonathan, who preferred being called Jon, lived in Crossman Hall—one of the Quad buildings—with two of his friends. As I strode down the litter-strewn hallway of Crossman, I averted my eyes from open doors. I never harbored masochistic tendencies and chose not to overwhelm my maternal sensibilities with visual assaults of trash and clothing that accumulated over the course of a semester. There was nothing I could do about the odors assailing my nose.

Jon greeted me at the door. Looking at him was like staring at an old Naval Academy midshipman photograph of his father. They had the same blue eyes, brown hair, and ruggedly handsome features. Of course, Bill's hair grayed right after our marriage. The timing of his graying pate was fortuitous and had nothing to do with his marriage to me—despite rumors to the contrary.

Jon graduated valedictorian of his high school class and entered the engineering department at CU. He had long known he would follow his father into some type of engineering. His love of computers—the bane of my existence—kept him challenged as a sophomore majoring in computer science.

Walking into Jon's room, I drank in the chaos affronting my eyes. I inhaled deeply, gagging on the unmistakable stench of dirty gym socks and stale beer. My eyes watered.

"Allergies acting up, Mom?"

I refused to answer the question on the grounds I might say something I'd regret later. "There's a lot of junk in here considering you've got to move out your stuff for Christmas, Jon. It doesn't look like you've packed anything."

"Funny, Mom. My roommates haven't left yet. It'll be straightened up before the room's inspected this afternoon."

I again feasted my tortured eyes on the three-man suite as Jon unceremoniously dumped clothes into a box. Straightening up the mess in a few hours would require an act of God.

"How do you find anything in this room? You've got piles of clothes, dishes, and books everywhere."

I couldn't see an inch of uncovered floor space. Okay, maybe that was an exaggeration. I spied a few cubic centimeters of stained carpeting. All three beds were heaped with junk. The walls were decorated with posters of beers and scantily clad women—pretty standard college room fare. I stared at a Twinkie nailed to the wall.

"Is that some kind of science project, Jon?"

"As a matter of fact, it is. We want to determine how long it remains in this pristine condition. Unfortunately, we'll have to remove it in June. Any chance I can continue the experiment at home?"

"Not a chance, Buster!" I laughed. I had my standards, although I lowered them to preserve peace at home. I didn't enter the children's rooms often. They kept their doors closed, so I was not constantly nauseated. The last time I peeked into Jon's room, I said a quick Hail Mary and shut the door.

I pointed to what I imagined were chairs under piles of clothes and books. "I'd love to rest my weary, aging bones, but I honestly can't see anywhere large enough for my butt."

Jon pointedly (in my opinion) ignored my comment. "Mom, all kidding aside, I appreciate you and Dad letting me work on papers at home. It's impossible accomplishing anything in the dorm. It's one party after another, and although they're fun, it's hard to concentrate."

I stared at him incredulously. "You expect me to believe that crap? Did I give birth to you? You must be one of only a handful of college students more concerned with schoolwork than parties."

He gave me a pitiful *I can't believe you don't believe me* look, but I wasn't to be fooled. I went to college after all. Truthfully, I enjoyed having Jon home, despite the tons of dirty laundry accompanying him. The mental picture of my laundry room when Jon was home reminded me of a question simmering on the back burner of my brain.

"If it's not too much trouble, Jon, I would like to know why clothes from the dorm smell so pungent."

"Well, you know how it is, Mom. We wear everything several times. I wear a shirt a couple of times right side out, then turn it inside out and wear it a couple more times. Same with underwear…"

"You can stop with the underwear, Jon. Unfortunately, I get the picture. My eyes water and my nose begs for congestion when I pass the washing machine on days you're home. As a matter of fact, the laundry room smells like the hallways here at Crossman. In case you're wondering, we do have enough money to buy more clothes."

"That's okay, Mom. We all smell the same after a while." He paused before saying, "You do know I'm joking about wearing my clothes inside out, don't you?"

"I'm not so sure about that, young man."

He stared at me, and although it shouldn't have made me uncomfortable, it did.

"Mom," he said quietly, "I need to talk to you. I've been trying to figure out how to ask this, but I haven't come up with any brilliant ideas, so here goes. Heather and I have been talking. She says you've been sort of quiet the past couple of weeks when she's home. I've noticed the same thing. Something's wrong. It isn't you and Dad, is it?"

"No, it's not your dad. He drives me crazy, but he's a good man. I have been self-absorbed lately, but I hoped to avoid mentioning my concerns until after Christmas. I'm sorry."

"Mom, Heather and I are worried. Rob seems oblivious, probably because he's rarely off the computer."

I took a minute to respond. I had not planned on dumping my personal crisis on my children, but Jon was an adult and entitled to an answer—an honest one.

"The day before Thanksgiving I felt a breast lump. I didn't worry about it, because I had a benign tumor removed from the other breast over twenty years ago. I had no palpable lymph nodes under my arm and decided it probably wasn't anything. I was overdue for a mammogram, so I called for an appointment. They squeezed me in the Friday after Thanksgiving. The mammogram looked okay to my untrained eye; at least I didn't see any big masses with stellate, uh—star-shaped—projections, which would have been ominous. Sorry, I'm rambling."

"It's okay, Mom. Please tell this your own way."

I felt choked up, knowing my son cared. I couldn't talk for several seconds. I took a deep breath. "The radiologist agreed that the films looked okay, Jon, but since I had a palpable lump, he ordered additional views, called compression views. An ultrasound to determine if the mass was a cyst followed the compression views. Those studies were done yesterday.

"After the ultrasound, I lay in that room staring at the ceiling for fifteen minutes before the technician returned with a radiologist. It seemed like an hour. A poster of Gabriel Byrne or Liam Neeson would have been nice to focus on. It was all I could do to keep from screaming, 'What did it show?' The radiologist repeated the ultrasound and then patted my arm; you know, the way I've told you nurses therapeutically touch patients. I remember thinking, 'I'm going to die.' "

Jon patted my arm. "Mom, I'm here for you, but if this is too much right now..."

I put my hand over his. "You've got that nice therapeutic touch down pat, buddy. Just like the radiologist."

Jon removed his hand. "I'm sorry you're going through this, Mom."

"I'm okay, Jon. I'm going to be fine." And at that moment, I really believed it. "Talking about this is difficult. I feel uncomfortable sharing feelings, but I'm touched you care enough to ask."

"I love you," he said quietly. "Does Dad know?"

"Nobody knows except the radiologist, ultrasound tech, and everyone I work with, since I see the docs in our office for care. I never thought I'd have to deal with something like this. I'm too healthy. My main risk factor is that I'm female. Of course, it doesn't help that I'm usually bombarded by stress at work and that I carried around nearly forty extra pounds of fat for several years."

"Does being overweight contribute to breast cancer, Mom?"

"It may. Fat seems to encourage estrogen to remain in the body longer, so cancers that are stimulated by estrogen…"

"Yeah. I get the picture, Mom. I really feel bad for you."

"Don't worry about me, kid. You know, it does bother me that if this is cancer, I will now be ground zero. Any woman in our family who gets breast cancer will look back at me and say, 'she started it,' even though I know more than eighty percent of breast cancer is not hereditary." I took another deep breath. "I'm digressing again."

"It's okay, Mom. I'm listening."

"I was left alone for another ten minutes while the radiologist called Dr. Bachelder. Everyone at work was waiting to hear about the outcome, so, with my blessing, she shared the news. She phoned last night and told me she had already made an appointment with a surgeon, Dr. Jones, for this morning. I laughingly asked, 'Does it look that bad?' She said the compression views showed a fixed area of architectural distortion with associated micro-calcifications, and the ultrasound was highly suspicious for malignancy."

"That sounds like Greek, Mom."

"It's just medical-ese for it doesn't look good."

"Oh."

"Of course, if I hadn't felt a mass, the compression views and ultrasound wouldn't have been done. My breast changes would have shown up on a regular mammogram at some point, but it wouldn't have been this year. I saw Dr. Jones this morning. He tried to move the lump away from the underlying tissue."

"What difference does it make if a lump is moveable, Mom?"

"If a breast mass is moveable, it isn't embedded in tissue or muscle. It's more likely to be a benign tumor, like a fibroadenoma. An immovable mass, which might include a tumor and the surrounding tissue's reaction, is more suspicious."

"Oh."

"Of course, it's not always easy telling the difference by feel alone. Dr. Jones thought it felt pretty moveable. He offered the option of a needle biopsy in his office, but he recommended removing the entire mass and sending it to pathology. I agreed to having the mass removed."

"I don't understand, Mom. What's a needle biopsy?"

"You are listening, aren't you?" I shot him a half smile. "After anesthetizing tissue, a needle is inserted into the mass—usually several times—and cells are extracted and sent to the lab for analysis. Both a needle biopsy and removal of the mass can determine if cancer exists. However, when one of the diagnostic tests shows a suspicious lesion, like my ultrasound did, it's probably more helpful to remove the entire mass. I decided to let Dr. Jones make the call."

"That was probably wise, Mom."

"I thought so. Where was I? I swear I'm starting to have brain farts."

"You decided to let Dr. Jones remove the whole thing."

"Right. Thanks. It must be wonderful to have a sharp, young brain. Dr. Jones sent in his amazing nurse, Joyce. Based on her conversation the day before with Dr. Bachelder, she had called the day surgery unit and tentatively set up my surgery for tomorrow, in case I wanted it; there had been an elective surgery cancellation. She even cleared it with our insurance company. Unbelievably, she did that in less than twenty-four hours. Insurance companies pay attention to the word cancer. So, tomorrow's the day."

"Wait a minute, Mom. You're having surgery tomorrow and you haven't told Dad?"

"I don't want to worry your dad, Jon. I'll be in and out of the hospital within a few hours, and I won't need to concern him if the tumor is benign. And if it's cancer, I'll share the bad news after Christmas. After all, by the time a woman finds a lump, it's been growing and spreading for several years. Some sources I've read indicate it takes eight to ten years before a mass is palpable—others indicate it might take less time for an aggressive tumor. Psychologically I can intellectualize this. Emotionally, I'm having difficulty accepting it."

"Mom, let's get home. You and Dad need to talk tonight. I know he'll want to go to the hospital with you. You're not thinking very clearly right now."

Chapter 3

"You look pooped, Pam," my husband, Bill, remarked. "Did you have a rough day?"

"I'd rather be at work than move Jon out of the dorm. You don't look so hot yourself." I hugged him. "Bad day at Rocky Flats?"

Bill collapsed on the couch. "Nothing went right today. Every time I turned around, someone called with another disaster. My day was reduced to crisis management and paper pushing. With all the restrictions, I'm surprised we accomplish anything. Cleaning up this plutonium mess is hard enough without being caught between Kaiser-Hill, the company overseeing this project, and the Department of Energy, which spins its wheels and ours introducing restrictions on a regular basis. Believe me, I do understand the need for protocols, but both groups regularly suggest conflicting methods for cleaning up the mess, and I spend countless hours in meetings reassuring both groups we can achieve our goals safely.

"Not only that, but the twentieth anniversary of the largest protest ever staged at Rocky Flats is coming up. It's amazing how times change. In the fifties, everyone was excited about the prospect of jobs the nuclear industry brought to this area. In the sixties, hippies staged countless sit-ins and demonstrations. Now they're protesting our plan to ship this radioactive stuff off site. What do they expect us to do with it? They have no idea what type of half-life we're talking about. You can't just let this stuff sit around, and it isn't like we haven't developed safe containers to encase the stuff. God, sometimes I really hate this job. I need time to relax awhile. Let me know if you need help making dinner."

When Bill was in a foul mood, which was rare, it was easier doing things myself, even though I despised cooking. I'd rather have ripped out my fingernails than bake a casserole, but I did it. Somebody had to.

"Mom!" Rob, my seventeen-year-old-son, shouted as he ran down the stairs. "I need $30 to reserve a copy of the yearbook." As a high school senior, Rob was 5'10" tall, thin, and handsome, with chestnut-brown hair and a perpetual smile. For the longest time, we could find no family member he resembled. The jokes ran the gamut of his being adopted to my having had an affair with the mailman, but I seem to remember the mailman being a woman around the time of his conception. My dad finally gave me a picture of my Opa (German grandfather) in his early twenties, and I swore

I was looking at Rob. So, at least we knew he belonged. Of course, since I remembered the delivery, I was fairly certain I was his mother—a woman who stands five-foot-two does not forget giving birth to a nine-and-a-half pound baby.

My daughter, Heather, once asked why we had three kids. Rob, who was Robbie until he let it be known he was too old to be called that, was unplanned, I told her. Rob, about six at the time, came to me in tears after his sister told him he was "a mistake". It took some time to convince my little angel that I hadn't phrased my comment that way. He weathered that traumatic revelation without too much permanent damage. He'd always been the family comedian, and I thought it appropriate that his due date was April 1st. Of course, he fooled us all and arrived the day before. Ever since, he'd maintained his status as the family's social leader. Girls called him all hours of the day and night. Bill finally put in a second phone line.

Sometimes he was too sociable. Notes and calls from his high school teachers testified to his being the class clown. "He is such an intelligent boy, Mrs. Stockho..." "If he would put as much effort into his schoolwork as he does learning jokes..." "If he'd do his homework..."

I tried! Honestly I did! Every gray hair on my head sprouted from my encouraging/begging/threatening that boy to take his studies seriously. In my heart, I knew Rob's education would be gained outside the classroom, and although an admirable comment to make about a child gifted in creating happiness for others, it was sometimes difficult to accept. Like so many of his generation, Rob taught himself to tame his computer. He became a whiz of a web designer, so I knew he could apply himself when motivated. I just couldn't motivate him to study what he needed to get into college.

Rob tried dragging me, kicking and screaming, into the computer age, but I resisted. I never embraced anything that couldn't yell back when I had issues. I screamed at my stupid computer and it invariably crashed—no warning, nothing. I could hold my own during a spirited two-way argument, but my computer consistently lost data, sent unfinished e-mails at random (no, I didn't touch the wrong button), and lacked compassion for mechanically challenged individuals like myself. It drove me crazy.

Rob gave me a peck on the cheek. "Mom, I've got to finish an article I'm writing for GameSpy. I'll see you later."

"Is there any hope you'll earn a few bucks from this gaming company, Rob?"

"I'm doing volunteer work, writing web news and articles for one of GameSpy's Web sites, Planet Shogo. It's so much fun, I don't care if I ever get paid."

That was my boy. His eyes would cross from spending years on that computer, and there wouldn't be a dime in it.

"Mom, where are you?" my twenty-one year old daughter called out. "I picked up a splinter in my finger from the deck and it hurts. That's what I get for brushing the dogs."

At 5'3 *and seven-eighths* inches, Heather towered over me by nearly two inches. Her light brown hair lightened to blond every summer, and her piercing blue eyes missed nothing. She was quite lovely, especially when she smiled. She worked hard keeping her trim figure. Rob inherited his Nana's skinny genes. The rest of us struggled.

Heather occasionally graced us with her presence. She was majoring in computers through the Business School at CU Boulder and lived near campus in an apartment Bill and I bought during her junior year. During the spring semester of her sophomore year, she'd worked at Walt Disney World in Orlando, as part of an exchange program through the School of Business. Heather had attended business seminars and worked as a lifeguard at the Wilderness Lodge Resort. When she returned to Boulder, dorm rooms for undergraduates, other than freshmen, were non-existent.

Heather loved outdoor sports, including skiing, snowboarding, swimming, and scuba diving. She hoped to pursue a career in resort management. For four years, she toiled at the CU pool, first as a lifeguard and then as assistant manager. Amazingly motivated, Heather sought out courses to improve her skills. In addition to her job, she taught CPR, swimming, and lifeguard training classes; assisted in scuba and aerobics classes; and babysat for several Louisville families.

I'd rarely seen a work ethic like hers. She worked too hard, but I tried not to tell her that too often. Heather thrived on pushing herself to excel. Sometimes I exhausted myself just thinking about her schedule.

"Hey, mom, where's the extra computer paper?" Jon bellowed from Bill's *I Love Me* room (aka the submarine memorabilia collected over twenty-four years of service in the United States Navy room). "I'm trying to print out info I downloaded, and we're out of paper." Cabinets banged. The noise drowned out some of his comments. The boy had only been home a few hours, and already the place reminded me of the monkey cage at the zoo. It would be a long Christmas break. Like the other men in my life, Jon rarely found anything without involving me.

The cacophony generated by three kids, three dogs, and a husband glued to the television set frequently challenged my sanity. Bill's channel flipping provided a background of constantly irritating babble that taxed any logical train of thought. "...The country fresh smell of...a dog sniffing your...sweaty underarms and feet...while you run along a deserted beach...drinking in forbidden pleasures...naked as the day you were born." Ah, life in the '90s.

Thinking about the needs of the children rather than the task of heating up potato soup for dinner, I tilted a glass pot as I pulled it out of a kitchen cabinet. Its lid crashed to the floor, shattering. I shooed the dogs away and dampened paper towels to clean up the mess.

"Rob, grab the checkbook from the desk in Dad's *I Love Me* room and ask him to write a check for your yearbook. Heather, look for the tweezers in the middle drawer in my bathroom cabinet. Betadine and band-aids are in the medicine chest. Jon, look in the cabinet to the right of the computer desk for the paper you need. And would it be too much to ask that the noise level in here be turned down a decibel or two?"

My own voice had an ear-splitting shrillness that drowned out the television. Not to be outdone by the children, the dogs competed for my attention. Holly, the oldest, bounced up and down, hoping someone would feed her.

"Not yet," Bill thundered from the family room. "It's still a half hour until your dinner time, Holly."

"Bill, do I make you wait when you're hungry?" I demanded as I filled Holly's bowl. As soon as dog food nuggets hit Holly's porcelain dish, the other canines raced into the kitchen.

At one time, I naively thought all golden retrievers were intelligent, but Holly constantly belied that supposition. As a puppy, she cheerfully de- voured rosebushes, complete with thorns. She pulled up floorboards and chewed carpeting. She ate plums dropping from trees until she was blessed with continuous diarrhea for weeks.

We shared our home with a second golden retriever, Hannah, who proved infinitely easier to train than Holly. With wagging tails and slobbery kisses, both dogs accosted everyone entering our homes.

Completing our canine menagerie was Heidi, a champagne-colored cocker spaniel with a lot of attitude. She was capriciously devoted to me.

According to Bill and the kids, Heidi sat by the front door for hours waiting for me to come home. As soon as I walked in, however, she immediately showed me her stump of a tail and ran for Bill's lap, giving me an *up yours* look. She had her routine: Bill's lap until bedtime and my feet for the night.

The dogs devoured their crunchy nuggets, while I heated up dinner for the rest of the household. Once upon a time, we ate dinner together, but rounding up high school and college-aged kids was like corralling sheep without a sheepdog. Sometimes Bill and I ate together, but I tended to forego much dinner, so he often plopped down in front of the television with a plate of food. Three canines ogled every forkful traveling from plate to mouth. Pathetic, soulful eyes and shoe-lace-long drool got their "we're still starving even though we ate ten minutes ago" point across. We weren't Ozzie and Harriet, but it worked for us.

The phone rang as I washed the dishes after dinner. It was my dear friend, Judy, calling from Virginia. Each of us claimed three kids, one Navy husband, and multiple military moves over the years. We attended graduate school together from 1984 to 1986. Leaning heavily on each other for emotional support during those two years, we laughed together, cried together, and saw each other more often than we did our families. Once, during our physical assessment class (where we practiced examining body parts on each other), I blurted out, "It's pretty pathetic when I see Judy naked more often than I do my own husband!" That had evoked lots of laughter, and no disagreement, from my classmates.

Judy and I endured the grueling, slave-driving hours of the nurse practitioner courses and clinicals, bitching only once or twice a day—the bitching was mostly mine. I was habitually sleep-deprived, because I want-ed to enjoy the children when I arrived home. Homework was completed after they were in bed. At times, I woke up the following morning asleep on one of the kids' beds. Bill never came looking for me, figuring his snoring drove me out of our bedroom. Looking back, I often wonder how I sur-vived. There truly must be guardian angels sitting on the shoulders of fools like me.

Actually, I know the guardian angel who helped me through that second flirtation with higher education. My mom drove up from North Carolina every week to stay with us from Monday through Friday. She chauffeured the kids to school, helped them with their homework, and made sure they ate better than I did when I stuffed my face with sodas and chips between classes. I couldn't have made it without her. Thanks, Mom!

"Pam, are you there?"

"Sorry, Judy. I was reminiscing."

"About what?"

"Graduate school."

I distinctly heard her groan.

"I should have known better than to tackle graduate school, Judy. The year before I was admitted, I took a statistics course and studied for the Graduate Record Exam for six months. One day Heather came home from Kindergarten with a picture of a nurse. The assignment had been to describe what a nurse does, and a teacher's assistant recorded the kids' answers. The teacher drew a big red question mark next to Heather's answer."

"What description did Heather give?"

"She said, 'A nurse is a lady who studies a lot and takes tests'."

Judy laughed.

Feeling maudlin, I remarked, "I never would have made it through school without you, Judy. At least, I *think* I'm grateful. Look how fulfilling our lives are now."

She snorted. "Feeling nostalgic tonight?"

"Yeah. It's great to hear your voice."

"Any exciting plans this evening, Pam?"

"I'm going to finish the dishes, and then burn off a couple hundred calories walking on my treadmill."

"You are so motivated."

"Not really. It's the only excuse I can come up with to watch movies and not feel guilty I'm avoiding household chores."

"Fun."

"Yeah. Usually."

"You sound down tonight. Anything bothering you?"

"I can't put anything past you, can I Judy?"

"Nope."

"I have a potential health problem."

"Anything you want to talk about, Pam?"

"Not yet. I'll let you know if anything devastating happens. It's just something on my mind for now."

"Okay, but let me know if you want to talk. Tell me what's going on in the great state of Colorado."

We talked for twenty minutes. We didn't solve any earth-shattering problems, but talking to Judy always raised my spirits. After I hung up the phone, I glanced over at Bill, still lounging in front of the television with Jon. I knew I should talk to him about my impending surgery, but I hadn't mustered up the courage. Jon looked over in my direction a couple of times; I knew what he was thinking. I shook my head and mouthed, "not now".

I studied my guys and smiled. In spite of the bustling activity with everyone home, I felt serene. Life had certainly changed from, "Please God, let me survive another six-month submarine deployment with three kids under the age of five and no family within three thousand miles!" to "I wonder when the kids will show up for a meal or a few bucks?" Life was easier, though Bill still rarely helped around the house.

A messy house never bothered him, but it drove me crazy. Bill snickered when I told him his helping around the house was a sexual turn on for me. Seeing him wash windows or vacuum got those juices flowing, but he never believed it. To his credit, he was willing to do anything I *asked him to do*. But it rankled me I had to ask. And yes, I urged him to notice the messes around him.

"Honey, honestly they don't bother me," he'd say. "Relax."

Sometimes I daydreamed. My daydreams were never about taking a lover—what real mom had time or energy for that? My dreams were more pragmatic. Yeah, they might involve another man, but he'd be cleaning my stove and refrigerator.

Bill was always a good sport about taking on occasional big jobs, though. In 1994, we bought a beautiful three-bedroom home in Louisville, knowing we'd have to add another bedroom in the basement to accommodate our family. Bill volunteered to undertake the job, and I've got to admit, he did an incredible job. He devoted almost two full years of downtime to the project. He completed all the electrical work, lighting, and drywall hanging. He put in a den, two bedrooms, a bathroom, and a large storage area, where I shimmied on my treadmill and lost myself in the escapades of Gabriel Byrne, Liam Neeson, Sean Connery, Peter O'Toole, Harrison Ford, or Tom Hanks.

I didn't watch a lot of movies or television otherwise. I generally preferred creating my own mental films while reading. Occasionally, I would pop a tape into the VCR at three in the morning, when I woke with a start, worried about a patient under my care. I averaged sleepless nights about three or four times a month. Watching some Hollywood stud prance across my screen was a lot more fun than staring at the ceiling for two hours. Sometimes, I'd get back to sleep afterwards, but I never counted on it. I wished I didn't worry so much. I was smart enough to know, for example, that kids with bacterial pneumonia would usually get better on antibiotics and wouldn't need hospitalization. Usually. However, it could be touch and go for the first thirty-six to forty-eight hours as their temperatures spiked, they were cranky, and parents' nerves frayed from lack of sleep. So *I* didn't sleep either.

After completing the basement, Bill swore that nothing on this earth could ever induce him to undertake such a monumental task again. We still bring visitors down to the basement so they can "Ooh" and "Ahh" over it. If you ever meet Bill, please mention the basement. He'll love you.

He did a lot of the work the first year in the house, when he and the boys moved out to Colorado alone. Yeah, that's right. Bill and the boys did the bachelor thing for nine months after Bill retired from the Navy and took the job at Rocky Flats in Colorado. Heather was approaching her senior year in high school in Virginia Beach, and understandably, she wanted to graduate with her friends. So for that school year, she, Heidi dog, and I lived in an apartment in Virginia Beach, while the fellows fended for themselves. They didn't starve, surviving on what Bill called his five-meal plan: fried chicken, Chinese take-out, macaroni and cheese, barbecued chicken, and pizza.

When Heather and I arrived for two weeks during Christmas break, the few fruits and vegetables in the crisper had developed a rainbow of colorful molds. There were tears in Bill's eyes. I had been truly missed. I spent two weeks cooking freezable casseroles and dinners, and for the first time in my life, I didn't bitch about cooking. I made up for other things besides cooking during those two weeks, but I'm leaving out the details.

During those interminably long nine months, Bill worked like a dog, finishing the basement so Heather would have a bedroom. He also taught in the Confirmation class, burning himself out in the parenting department. I thought the experience might change his attitude about helping around the house, but by the time Heather graduated, he was ready to slip back into his complacent "let things slide, honey" mood.

I swear that as we packed the U-Haul to bring Heather and me to Colorado, I cried. "I don't want to go," I sobbed.

I'd had such a lovely nine months, with time for myself and time to make photo albums for the kids for Christmas from the boxes of pictures I'd never organized. Of course, my reticence to move made Bill feel like crap.

And I felt bad, but just a little. I finally pulled myself together, and we journeyed westward. I soon fell in love with Colorado.

Wonderful neighbors hastened my love of the state. I regularly saw them when I worked outside in the yard. Mind you, they only showed up at very specific times. If I was decked to the nines in some cute little outfit I paid too much for, they were nowhere to be seen. However, if I figured I'd get one last wearing out of the faded, ripped T-shirt I got from the kids for Christmas sporting something like a "Mamma, you the man!" logo, coupled with a pair of jeans with a hole in the seat that didn't quite cover my half-off sale Jockey floral bikini briefs, they'd all be out to say hello. It was okay. I caught them in equally embarrassing states.

Our home was only two miles from the Louisville Family Medical Center. I couldn't believe my good fortune in living so close to my job. I occasionally walked home when my car was on the fritz and the child who was supposed to pick me up failed to make an appearance. I didn't mind. The exercise was good for me.

I loved being a family nurse practitioner. I loved the staff at our clinic, especially the nurses, who regaled me with ribald jokes, which I immediately passed on. I treated many of my patients as extended family members. Living in a small town was great. I ran into friends and patients at the supermarket, hairdresser, and library. I had almost everything a woman could want, and I counted myself blessed. I had wonderful kids and a pretty great husband (a few points off in the helping out around the house department, but otherwise not bad at all—definitely a keeper).

As I finished reflecting about my good fortune, I smiled once more at Jon and Bill sharing a television moment. I turned and plodded back into the kitchen. Suddenly my cheerful mood vanished. I desperately wanted to enjoy loads more time with my children and husband. "Please God, don't let this be cancer. I promise I won't ask anything for myself ever again. Please!" I bent over the sink and sobbed.

Jon noticed. He walked into the kitchen and hugged me. "Talk to Dad, please."

My jumbled thoughts derailed, and I vainly attempted to drive the train wreck of pathetic, feel-sorry-for-myself thoughts from my mind. "I will, Jon. A little later, but I promise I will."

I would talk to Bill about the surgery before we went to bed, but I was feeling too sorry for myself to discuss it before that. I headed down to the basement to walk on my treadmill.

Chapter 4

My walk invigorated me and lifted my mood. I wasn't sure if my improved outlook was due more to exercise-induced endorphins or watching Gabriel Byrne in *The Man in the Iron Mask*, but either way, I was grateful for the attitude adjustment. After my shower, I talked to Bill about my impending surgery.

"Why you?" Bill demanded when I dropped my bomb.

Why indeed? I thought. I had no answers. Bill was glad that I mentioned it. He called his boss, whose wife had weathered her own scare with a breast lump (a false alarm). Per his boss, Bill would not be expected at work in the morning.

I was relieved after sharing my worrisome burden. There had been so many years when I hadn't shared concerns with him—mainly the years submarines took him to sea. I learned to rely on myself, like other Navy wives. We wives talked amongst ourselves, and many of us became very close friends as a result, but it wasn't the same as talking to the men we'd chosen to spend our lives with—the partners we looked to for guidance, companionship, and romance. Having Bill home consistently was the greatest benefit of his retiring from the Navy, but I was still reticent to dump my fears on him.

Unable to sleep, I lay in bed and stared at the ceiling, drawing on past coping strategies to ease my anxiety. Relax. Breathe in; breathe out. God's up there somewhere. God will help. Faith had gotten me through many tough situations, although my views about the Catholic Church had radically modified through the years. Pulling the covers up to my shoulders, I reflected on my religious metamorphosis. As a child, neither I, nor my peers, ever questioned the authority of priests and nuns, although much about their discipline left me with conflicted emotions.

I still got a bit clammy thinking about nuns walking between rows of desks, their rosary beads clacking as they moved. They rarely smiled. Rulers in their hands were used to rap knuckles of inattentive students. I grew up afraid of Sisters, wondering why women supposedly so devoted to God harbored such readiness to inflict corporal punishment. Thankfully, I rarely endured that punishment. I kept out of trouble by memorizing the Baltimore Catechism, learning my prayers, and vomiting back memorized answers to questions posed.

On the other hand, I had fond memories of Father Lynch, the jovial Oblate of Mary Immaculate priest who presided over St. Ann's Church and guided the students of the associated Catholic school. No matter how stern he tried to be during his catechism lectures, the twinkle in his eye always gave him away. He preferred the occasional pat on the head for answers correctly given. I remember his being the bane of the principal's existence the year I was in eighth grade.

"You're undoing all we've accomplished with strict discipline," Sister chided him once when I had kitchen duty cooking the nuns' lunches. "You let them get away with murder, Father. Those children know they'll just get a warning when they misbehave, and their unacceptable behavior will be encouraged by a little laugh from you."

"Now, Sister," he began as the two of them left the kitchen, "surely you can remember being a bit rambunctious when you were young."

"Never!" Sister adamantly protested.

"She's probably right," my friend, Denise, muttered, stirring gravy. "She probably came into this world, ruler in hand, screaming, 'Let me at those rotten little monsters!'"

"Shush!" I scolded. "She'll be back in here to take a switch to our legs."

"Let her. I'll put ex-lax in the gravy."

The memory cheered me. Bill let out an earsplitting snore, and I nudged him onto his side. The man could wake the neighbors two houses down the way he sawed logs. I'd worn earplugs nightly since the children were old enough to find me if they experienced a nightmare or needed a drink of water.

I thought again of Father Lynch, his nicotine-stained fingers and constant hacking cough a reminder of his two-pack a day cigarette habit. He died from lung cancer in his early sixties.

Bill smoked about a pack a day, despite my begging him to quit. I'd often chided him, asking if his insurance policies were paid up, wondering aloud if he wanted to make me a young widow with three small children. My nagging made no difference, so I stopped wasting my breath and making him feel guilty. He loved me, but he would only quit when he was ready. I sometimes wondered if he would meet the same fate as Father Lynch, dead before his time from cancer. But I couldn't talk, could I? I might be facing the same fate.

I didn't know if Father Lynch was buried in the small graveyard across the street from St. Ann's Church. I'd often visited the cemetery after school, pausing over the many graves of local Civil War veterans. Around each Memorial Day, I read and lingered over each name decorated with a flag.

Cemeteries always comforted me, as morbid as that may sound. I think my solace grew naturally from my past. As young children, my sister and I pushed our baby doll carriages through rows of ornate headstones in the cemetery across from the apartment building where we lived with our parents in Munich, Germany. Dad, who was born in Germany, returned there as an officer in the U.S. Army in the early 1950's.

Magnificent marble statues of angels and saints stood guard over graves throughout the grounds of our beautiful German cemetery. Peace enveloped me as Linda and I walked among them. The only sound disturbing our reverie was the scraping of the carriage wheels along the gravel. Adults perpetually resting there never told me to put dishes in the sink, pick up my toys, be quiet, answer when spoken to, or finish my vegetables because there were starving babies in Africa and China who would be grateful for the food left on my plate. Those admonitions came from the maids who worked for my parents.

My captivation with cemeteries continued. In high school, one of my favorite books was the *Spoon River Anthology*, by Edgar Lee Masters, a story about a town told by its deceased inhabitants in the form of epitaphs. Every base the Navy assigned Bill to felt more like home once I wandered among the local graveyards.

My favorite cemeteries boasted humorous epitaphs. That's probably where my morbid sense of humor originated. I discovered the best ones in Connecticut. I thought it ironic that the droll wit of epitaphs so sharply contrasted with the stark reserve I observed in many New Englanders.

My eyelids fluttered. Exhaustion invaded every cell, but sleep eluded me. I feared that closing my eyes and clearing my mind would allow cancer to creep into my thoughts. I chased ideas of illness from my consciousness by thinking of another parish, of another time.

I attended college at Virginia Commonwealth University in Richmond and had the fortuitous advantage of living in a dormitory two blocks from the archdiocese's cathedral. Its architecture reminded me of the elaborate German churches I treasured as a child. I loved its gilding and exquisitely crafted stained glass windows. Rows of vigil candles, lit by those in need of saintly intercession, graced both sides of the altar rail. Occasionally, I left an offering and lit one of the white candles, praying I would master a test. I would watch the flame glow eerily through the crimson candleholder and feel guilt for having lit a candle for my miserably banal concern. For my penance, I would read for a few extra hours to blind students who depended on the kindness of others to get through their textbooks. Of course, I never minded reading to the blind; I never turned down any excuse to read.

Half asleep, my hazy mind continued to drift while Bill's snoring penetrated my thoughts. I'd occasionally heard such window rattling recitals in church, usually when a priest droned on during homilies. Although I didn't sleep during Mass, I'd often been guilty of allowing my thoughts to wander. Focusing on the priest had sometimes been at the heart of my inattentiveness, especially when I was a college coed. Father *What-a-Waste* was a priest at the cathedral in Richmond during the early 1970s. With jet-black hair framing his incredibly handsome face, he attracted a bevy of female undergraduates to his Masses. We all thought it a miserable waste that he should remain celibate when so many of us would gladly have borne his children. I spent more than a few hours confessing to impure thoughts about "a man".

Even though the Catholic Church and I disagreed more with each passing year, there were lingering beliefs I couldn't dismiss. In spite of my less than stellar behavior in following the precepts of my church—I went to Mass frequently, but not every Sunday, for instance, and I didn't believe I'd go to hell as a result—I hoped I'd be lucky enough to have a priest around just before the end, so I could make a deathbed confession. However, a dearth of vocations to the priesthood and a steady efflux of men wishing to marry meant the odds of having a priest around before I faced St. Peter were not in my favor.

If the Church elevated women to the priesthood and allowed priests to marry and live within the warm embrace of families, problems of recruitment might evaporate. I could only imagine the difficulties inherent in lifelong celibacy. Disclosures of physical abuses of altar boys and others entrusted to the care of religious men and women frequently tore at my heart.

While on my wayward path of expounding on opinions regarding the faith I embraced at Baptism, I probably sealed my fate by espousing birth control. Forbidding birth control never prevented sex—big news flash, right? But the Church hierarchy never accepted that. Their disavowing the importance of condoms in this world of rampant sexually transmitted diseases, including many for which there remained no cure, was reckless and dangerous. God help me, but I always thought it a terrible impertinence that men sat in luxury in Rome, their every need fulfilled, while they dictated the way people should live their lives in poverty and suffering, bringing into this world more children than they and the earth could sustain. Yeah, I'd heard the saying, "God will provide", but I preferred, "God helps those who helps themselves", and for me, that included taking responsibility to prevent unwanted births and sexually transmitted diseases.

I always believed I would never consider abortion as a personal choice, but through the years, I counseled too many rape and incest victims to irrevocably believe that I would not have sought relief from the mental and physical anguish such acts cause. As I aged, my absolutely solid, "I firmly believe", "no way will I ever change my mind" principles became less tenable. That didn't mean I no longer felt strongly about many subjects, but I came to believe that others' opinions were as important and deserving of respect as mine, as long as they didn't involve harming others. And I understood that harming others depended on one's perspective about when life began and ended.

My mind worked in strange and mysterious ways when I was tired, especially when I was avoiding confronting personal crises. During those times, it was easier solving world problems than facing decisions that impacted my personal little life. Drifting towards REM sleep, I could convince myself that all we needed to change the world were leaders who would put the concerns of the needy above those of big business, big spenders, and big campaign contributors. The night before my first breast surgery was definitely at the top of my "let's see what world crises I can solve without venturing into the more frightening world of Pam's problems" list. I tried in vain to ignore Bill's snoring echoing off the walls. I desperately needed sleep, but I became increasingly nervous as the night dragged on. The results of the morning's biopsy could change my life radically. As much as I complained about wanting a change, cancer was not the one of which I dreamed.

Chapter 5 - December 18th

I handed my insurance card to the day surgery receptionist at Boulder Community Hospital and numbly answered questions I couldn't remember two minutes later. To be honest, I was barely cognizant of my surroundings, but the soothing sound of a waterfall filtered through. A gentle cascade of water trickled melodiously down the surface of an abstract mountain etched out of roughly hewn rocks. I concentrated on its tranquilizing sound to impede images of my impending surgery. Despite Bill's reassuring presence, I felt alone.

The receptionist smiled frequently, but I shivered. My mind blanked as we walked to the waiting area. Bill and I had shared twenty-three years, half my life, and I could think of nothing to say. I sat among other frightened, silent people—or perhaps my perception was merely a projection of my fear.

Bill kneaded my hand. Alone with my few fleeting thoughts, I summoned up the conversation Bill and I had shared the night before. Lying in bed, he'd held my hand and grasped for comforting words; he really had. Little had penetrated my rising anxiety. It was all right. Absorbing his consoling phrases wouldn't have changed the fact I hadn't slept a wink the entire night, but his concern warmed my heart.

"Pam," he'd said before drifting off to sleep, "since you're a nurse, I know you understand what we're facing. I want you to know that's how I think of this situation—as something we're facing together. I haven't always been around during crises. Being in the Navy meant frequent separations, but I was really proud of you. You organized everything so well. Sometimes I felt like a fifth wheel—as if the family fit me in for the few weeks I was home." He'd squeezed my hand again. "I haven't been very helpful at home either."

I felt like a priest, hearing confession. "I didn't know you felt you didn't belong, Bill."

"It wasn't so much that as it was knowing the children didn't accept discipline from me when they were young. They rarely came to me when they were hurt or had questions. I didn't want to complain, especially since you were stuck with them most of the time."

"I love the kids. I never felt stuck with them, although I was often exhausted." I'd laughed. "Okay. That's a little exaggeration. Sometimes I begged for relief from three rug rats who needed constant supervision. Remember your unexpected transfer from Connecticut to San Diego a couple of weeks after Robbie was born? I had hives for the five months you were at sea. They disappeared the day you returned. I loved submarine homecomings. You planned great adventures. The children saw you as a plaything rather than a disciplinarian. As a matter of fact, I enjoyed the playing around as well."

"I'm glad you did, Pam, but I wish you could have counted on me. When we moved every two or three years, you four unpacked the boxes, made new friends, and found schools, vets, and doctors. Then I'd come home from sea to a house unpacked and set up."

"Except for the pictures. I always left those for you to hang."

"Except for those."

"It wasn't a piece of cake for you either, Bill, under the ocean for weeks or months at a time with guys who probably didn't bathe much and who spent too much time in the bathroom, excuse me, *the head*, reading *Playboy* articles."

"There were some great articles in *Playboy*."

"I'll bet. *Playboy* is an important literary source for men, isn't it?"

"It is. And the jokes; don't forget the jokes, Pam."

"Of course not. The jokes. They must be hilarious, and I'm sure a main motivating factor in sailors' buying the magazine." He laughed and so did I. "Thanks, Bill, I need that."

"You're welcome. I love your smile, Pam, and I'll love you no matter what happens. I want you to know that."

I loved him at that moment more than I ever had. "That means more to me than you will ever know."

"Since I'm unloading tonight, may I continue, Pam? I feel like I'm going to confession."

"Ah, I was thinking the same thing. Just so you don't turn the table on me, asking for my confession and giving me last rites."

"Don't even joke about that. I can't live without you."

What could I say to that?

"Pam, if you have cancer, you'll need my help. I'll be there for you."

I appreciated those sentiments the night before, and they still made me smile. I forced my attention to the present and my pending surgery. I looked at Bill.

"Pam, I'm sorry," he said. "I've been lost in thought. I should be comforting you."

"That's okay, Bill. I don't feel like talking. I'm just glad you're here." He kissed my cheek. "And thanks again for last night."

"Which part? The confession part or the forcing you out of your own bed because of my snoring part?"

I smiled.

"Pamalla Stockho," a cute young nurse called from the entrance to the surgical suite.

My heart beat faster. "How come everyone in the world looks young today, and I feel like a withered old prune?"

"You're the best looking prune I've ever seen," Bill said.

"Life isn't fair." I rose from my seat. "I've lost thirty-eight pounds, patients tell me how great I look, and NOW I may have breast cancer?"

"You look gorgeous, as beautiful as the day I met you."

"You're full of shit, but thanks, I needed that."

"You take compliments SO well, my dear."

We followed the nurse past several cubicles—tiny spaces with room only for a gurney and small chair—until she stopped at one marked with my name. I shivered. A flimsy curtain provided a modicum of modesty as I removed my clothing. I don't know why I bothered, but I carefully folded each item, placing everything but my eyeglasses, socks, and underwear in a plastic bag that bore my name.

After putting on a thin, cotton, hospital gown and climbing onto the gurney, the pre-op nurse put on my armband and started an IV. Since I was shivering like I was standing in the middle of an iceberg butt-naked, my sympathetic and observant nurse placed a warm blanket over me.

"Dr. Jones will arrive shortly to obtain a pre-op history and do a physical exam," she told me. "You'll go into surgery in about an hour. Dr. Jones left orders we could provide anti-anxiety medication if you need it. Would you like some now?"

"No, thank-you," I told her. "I'd feel better keeping a clear head. I'll let you know if I need anything."

"Okay. It's funny how differently women face these breast surgeries. Some are so freaked out they insist on being put out completely. And others, like yourself, don't want anything at all."

"We're all different, I guess. How long will it be from the start of surgery until I can go home?"

"The surgical prep and procedure take about forty-five minutes to an hour, and then you'll return here to recover," my nurse said. "If you only have a local anesthetic, we'll obtain a set of vital signs and discharge you within a few minutes."

Waiting for Dr. Jones, I said nothing. I didn't want to worry Bill unnecessarily, although I felt increasingly apprehensive. Part of my apprehension was the realization I could do nothing to influence the results of my biopsy. The thought disquieted me. For the first time since I'd begun practice as a nurse, I envisioned myself as a patient. I pictured myself sitting across from my mirrored image in a small examination room. The fear I'd observed in patients waiting for test results flooded my eyes. I'd held many who cried after hearing devastating news. My gut wrenched and my chest hurt for their pain. But I'd never been able to empathize with them—until this moment.

Dr. Jones' smiling face intruded upon my morbid thoughts. I smiled uncertainly at Bill. After the surgeon completed his exam, he said, "We'll be ready to move you over to surgery in about thirty minutes. Do you have any final questions, Pam?"

"Last requests" was how my pathetic mind interpreted the remark. "When will we know the pathology results, Dr. Jones?"

"We'll have a preliminary report on the biopsied tissue before you leave today. I'll be in to see you after you return here to recover. One of the nurses will show you to the waiting room, Mr. Stockho. She'll look for you there after your wife's surgery is completed."

"Why don't you get some lunch, Bill?" I suggested as Dr. Jones walked away. "There's no reason we should both starve. Actually, I'm too upset to eat, but I don't think I've ever been so thirsty."

"Okay, I'll go to McDonald's. I'll be back in about an hour. Love you." He kissed me.

Time dragged once Bill left. Quietly waiting, I reflected on our clinic patients who were battling breast cancer. I most admired Beth Heston, a thirty-three year old mother of two—Thomas, age eight, and Barbara, age four. Beth had come to me after finding a breast lump. The mass felt firm and fixed to the underlying tissue, but because of her young age, I hoped the tumor would be benign.

"But we have to be certain," I'd told her. "I'll schedule a mammogram for you, although until about age thirty-five, breast tissue is so dense it may be difficult to identify an underlying tumor. Since mammogram results may not be definitive, I will also schedule an ultrasound to determine if this is a cyst."

Two days later, the radiologist confirmed a very suspicious mass by ultrasound.   Surgical lumpectomy corroborated the earlier suspicion, the mass an infiltrating ductal carcinoma by pathology, a "garden variety" breast cancer, as the surgeon had pointed out. Beth's reaction to everything that ensued was inspirational. She bought a wig when her hair fell out from chemotherapy, and she continued to care for her children despite overwhelming fatigue that plagued her through both chemotherapy and radiation.

"I smile as much as I can," she told me. "That doesn't mean I never feel sorry for myself, but I keep going for my husband and the children." Now, several months after the completion of treatments, her hair showed signs of growth, and the fatigue was slowly waning.

"God," I begged, "please let me be as brave as Beth if this is cancer."

...

"Why do gurneys, like grocery carts, always have at least one wheel that wobbles?" I wondered aloud as my nurse steered the tortuous path past other gurneys and carts obstructing the hallway to the operating room. The temperature hovered around freezing in the operating room—at least it felt that way under my alluring cotton patient's gown. Three pairs of hands lifted and pulled me onto the table.

"Hi, Pam," a friendly voice said. "My name is Dan Martin. I'm a registered nurse, trained in conscious sedation. I probably won't be needed much today, but I'll monitor your vital signs and give you medications if you feel anxious during the procedure. I've got lots of good stuff, so don't hesitate to say something if you're feeling the least bit nervous. We're going to put a large drape in front of your face, but I'll let you know what happens every step of the way. We're going to secure both of your arms at about ninety degrees from your body. That will enable us to access your IV easier, allow us to monitor your blood pressure and oxygen saturation, and also prevent you from helping Linda here, who will spend the next five minutes or so washing the surgical area with nice warm Betadine. Ready?"

My teeth chattered as my gown was removed from my chest.

"Yo, let's have some warm blankets for the lady freezing to death under this drape," Dan ordered. "Pam, we'll have you covered as much as

39

possible when Linda finishes scrubbing your breast." Dan turned to face the operating room door, as it swung open, and proclaimed with flair, "Ah, the great surgeon arrives. Hey, Ralph, how about a little disco music?"

I asked Dan (the only face I could see in the sterile environment), "Doesn't the surgeon pick the music?"

"Heck, no." He chuckled. "That only happens in the movies. You think he rates around here?"

"That's right, I get no respect around here," said Dr. Jones. "At least my patients love me."

"That's 'cause they don't know you like we do, doc," Ralph guffawed.

I tried to keep my sense of humor throughout the exchange, although I felt uneasy. "Uh, Dan, is there something I should know as the patient before my doctor carves me up like a Thanksgiving turkey?"

"No, Dr. Jones is fabulous. We just give him a hard time because we can. Ladies and gentlemen, we're making the patient nervous. Shall we get started?"

Dr. Jones peeked around the drape. "Don't worry, Pam. They're just jealous because I make the big bucks."

"Yeah, right!" they yelled in unison.

"Pam, Dr. Jones will infiltrate the surgical area with a local anesthetic," Dan said. "Then, he'll make an incision just below the mass and remove it, along with some surrounding tissue. You may feel tugging and hear hissing as he uses a cautery to stop the bleeding."

A couple of times during the procedure, I felt sharp, stabbing pain as Dr. Jones sliced at tissue not fully anesthetized. Each time, Dan, acutely aware of my grimaces, requested additional anesthetic before I could even comment on my discomfort. I became nauseated as I realized that the smell of flesh being cauterized was my own. I tried to keep up a repartee with Dan, although I didn't feel particularly witty.

"I can't think of a single joke to tell you, Dan, and I can usually come up with a bunch."

"That's okay, Pam. This is probably not the easiest thing you've gone through." He told me about his move from California the previous year, because he wanted his children to grow up in a safe area. His wife enrolled at CU to earn a degree in early childhood education. We commiserated on the CU Buffs' miserable football season and the hope the team would improve during the next year. Before I knew it, I was wheeled back to recovery. Thank God for caring nurses!

Bill arrived twenty minutes later. He looked frustrated. "I was told to wait in the surgical waiting room, but your nurse looked for me in the day surgery waiting room. I'd still be there if I hadn't wandered in here looking for you. I was beginning to worry. It took longer than I expected."

"Sorry for the confusion, Bill. Now if we just receive good news from pathology…" Bill kissed me. My nurse wrapped a blood pressure cuff around my right arm.

The look on Dr. Jones' face forced acid into my throat. A squeezing chest pressure prevented me from taking a deep breath.

"It appears to be an infiltrating ductal carcinoma," Dr. Jones said. "It's the most common type of breast cancer. Of course, we have to wait for the final pathology report, and I know you won't take in a lot of what I say, but I'll go over this again when you come into the office in about a week."

He was talking to me. I saw his lips move. But what was he saying? Cancer? Impossible! I'd always been healthy. Oh, God! I loosened my death grip on Bill's hand. My stomach knotted. Don't fall apart! Don't fall apart in front of Bill, I screamed at myself. There's got to be some mistake. My eyes clouded with tears. How will I get through this? How does one deal with being told the life you've taken for granted may end? Oh sure, people die every day—but I don't. Not me. I have so much to do.

Incredibly, the only thoughts that popped into my mind at that moment were of two books I'd recently read: *1916* by Morgan Llywelyn and *Irish Hunger* by Tom Hayden. The books covered two periods of history when the Irish people fought for their lives and their culture. It made absolutely no sense to me that I would think of Ireland at that moment. After all, I had no ties to that tiny island country. I had been reading Irish history only to understand a little about the culture from which some of my favorite actors came—nothing more. But somehow, focusing on what others had suffered eased my anxiety. I think we called it displacement in psychology class years ago.

Dr. Jones was still talking. "You have a lot to think about, Pam and Bill. In a couple of weeks, I'll perform a second surgery to remove lymph nodes from under your arm to determine if the cancer has spread to your lymph system. The prognosis is about the same whether you have a lumpectomy or a mastectomy for this type of cancer, as long as you receive the recommended post-surgical treatments. In the event you opt for a lumpectomy, I may need to dissect additional tissue if the margins of the tumor removed today aren't clear of cancer. If you choose to have a mastectomy, reconstructive surgery can either be done at the time of surgery or you may have it done later. Reconstruction is now completely covered by insurance.

"You and your husband need to discuss your options and let me know your decision. You can take a week or so to think about this, but it would be best for the second surgery to take place before the end of the year. I'm sorry. I know this will spoil your Christmas." He paused, and his kind eyes settled on me. "Before you leave today, I will order blood work, an EKG, and a chest X-ray. Please call my office Monday to schedule a follow-up appointment. Do you have any questions?"

"Just one." I choked back tears. My voice cracked. "After the next surgery, what's the usual treatment for this type of cancer?"

"Your oncologist will review all of that when you make an appointment with him, but the standard of care for such a young woman as yourself is six rounds of chemotherapy followed by five weeks of radiation, if you choose the lumpectomy."

After Dr. Jones left, Bill stared blankly at me. "I know you probably understood what he was saying, but I'm in the dark. Why do you need another surgery?"

I took a deep breath. Keep it together, Pam, I told myself. Keep it together. I was afraid that if Bill saw me fall apart, he would too. I willed myself to open my mouth and answer. I responded in the only way I could and keep from crying; the clinical nurse practitioner spit out information like a robot.

"The lymph nodes under the armpit are the drainage system for the breast, Bill. Removing nodes gives the surgeon and oncologist a better idea of whether or not this has spread extensively. If cancer has spread to the lymph nodes, it's much more likely the cancer has already seeded elsewhere. He will also need to reopen the incision he made today if the tissue that was removed doesn't have clear margins. That would mean cancer tissue still remains in my breast."

"If he does the second surgery and gets all the cancer, why do you have to have chemotherapy and radiation treatments?"

"The answer to that is more difficult." I willed myself to fight the nausea I felt. This is me I'm talking about. Not some character in a book. Bill watched me, his eyes two huge question marks. I swallowed with difficulty.

"Tumors like this (I couldn't say 'mine') have been growing for several years by the time a lump is large enough to palpate. Blood vessels to the tumor grow rapidly and are pretty impressive. Believe me, as much burning as I smelled during his cauterization of blood vessels, I am able to attest to the tumor's having a great blood supply."

I stopped, momentarily unable to go on. The nausea worsened. I cleared my throat. "A good blood supply allows cancer cells to enter the blood stream and invade other organs. The aim of chemotherapy is to destroy those cancer cells. Various classes of chemotherapeutic agents interfere with different phases of cell reproduction, so several meds are used. Unfortunately, healthy dividing cells are also affected. That's why one gets side effects from chemotherapy like nausea, vomiting, mouth ulcers, and hair loss, as well as depletion of cells that fight infection and prevent bleeding." I forced the disquieting image from my mind.

"Although Dr. Jones will excise all the cancerous tissue he can find, abnormal cells may remain. Radiation kills cells locally, but the radiation used does not destroy large areas of cells. If that much radiation were used, healthy tissue would also be destroyed, if it didn't kill the patient. There are no guarantees, Bill. Even if I have a mastectomy, cancer has been known to come back in the surgical scar. And if by some miracle all of the cancer is removed with the surgery, I'll be taking an unnecessary risk with chemo-therapy and radiation."

"What do you mean?"

I sighed. "Both chemotherapy and radiation may cause cancer, Bill. The probability is small, but the risk has to be considered." Considered— how very analytical of me. I didn't want to die—not yet. Please! "However, the aim of combining therapies is to reduce the risk of recurrence. It's a crapshoot, Bill. And I'm not sure yet what I want to do. We need to talk when I'm feeling less despondent." I mustered a small smile. "Right now I want to go by the liquor store and buy a bottle of Asti Spumante. You can help me polish it off. I don't want to think anymore today. Just for a while, I want to numb any emotion."

Chapter 6 - December 24th

Six days after surgery, I experienced another morbid attack of self-pity. I chose to curl up on the couch rather than spend a couple of hours at the mall with Bill and the kids. I desperately needed to extract myself from the spiraling pit of despair I'd created, a place where I'd wallowed intermittently since surgery.

I sipped a glass of white zinfandel. I only drank occasionally, but those occasional times had occurred almost nightly since the words *cancer* and *me* became irrevocably entwined. A pitiful, strangled laugh escaped my lips. I found it difficult, and at times impossible, to reconcile myself to the fact which so unceremoniously slapped me in the face: you've got cancer, baby. Deal with it. I didn't want to deal with it. I didn't want to deal with anything. This could be my last Christmas.

Instead of talking to Bill about my escalating anxieties, I bottled my fears and let them suffocate me. Great therapy. I feared death and wanted to verbalize it, but Bill felt uncomfortable with any reference to dying. I didn't want to burden friends. I could have joined a support group, but I knew I'd fall into the role of health care provider, trying to comfort everyone else. I wasn't ready to deal with others' fears. Oh well. I had managed when Bill was at sea for months at a time, and I could do it again.

Despite my desire to protect them from raw, uncensored emotions, my friends were wonderful. There were many phone calls. "I'm sorry this happened to you." "Can I bring over dinner?" "Do you need anything?" "You're so brave." The bravura was a well-played act. My emotions were as tightly wound as a fiddle string ready to snap.

As ridiculous as it sounds, I still hoped for that impossible phone call: "Mrs. Stockho, we're so sorry. The pathologist took another look at your biopsied tissue and there is no cancer. We apologize for any emotional pain and inconvenience we might have caused…"

Denial, denial. My mind sifted through twenty-three years of nursing service. I'd always claimed a fabulous immune system. I rarely developed the snotty-nosed, "slimy green stuff like pus sliding down my throat—wanna see?" illnesses which patients described in nauseating detail.

Suddenly, the irony that I had cancer struck me as hysterical. When I needed my immune system the most—when that first cancer cell escaped destruction by phagocytes—it had failed me. I laughed out loud, but the laughter quickly disintegrated into choked sobbing.

Heidi cautiously padded her way to my side, her little cocker stump wagging furiously. Hesitantly, she pawed at my leg, gazing up worriedly at my tear-streaked face. I smiled at her. Encouraged, she took a tentative jump into my lap, missed, and crashed to the floor. She barely missed hitting her head on the coffee table. I scooped her into my arms. "Don't worry about me, girl."

Holly and Hannah lingered nearby. Their tails beat the carpet savagely while their eyes trained on my face. Ah, the unconditional love of furry friends!

I focused on the Christmas tree across the room. Standing, I crossed to it and caressed ornaments collected from the journeys we'd made as a family—trinkets representing key events. There were submarines created from dough, felt, and glass, each engraved with the boat number to which Bill had been assigned. Wooden knickknacks reminded me of national parks where we camped and vacationed. All the dogs who'd shared our lives were pictured: Tigger, Penny, Holly, Hannah, and Heidi. Each city we had lived in and loved was immortalized: Groton, Connecticut; Portsmouth, New Hampshire; Kittery, Maine; San Diego, California; Virginia Beach, Virginia; Mare Island, California; Gales Ferry, Connecticut; and Louisville, Colorado. Some of the cities were depicted twice—once for each Navy tour.

I fingered the baubles that held my children's pictures and chronicled their loves: swim team, little league, Cub Scouts, Boy Scouts, Brownies, Girl Scouts, gymnastics, ballet, life guarding, skiing, snowboarding, aerobics, hiking, camping, bicycling, and rafting.

Kneeling, I touched the priceless pieces handmade by Heather, Jon, and Rob. Tradition dictated hanging those decorations on lower branches, within easy reach, even when the children all surpassed me in height.

There were so many ornaments it was difficult to see them individually any more. I stepped back. All those separate memories made a whole—the Stockho legacy—Bill's and my dreams realized in our children. In that single sentimental moment, I realized how miraculous my life had been so far—so far. My life wasn't close to being over. I vowed to fight.

I retraced my steps, sat down on the couch, and picked up my glass of wine. I sipped slowly, dwelling on a past held forever captive in tiny bits of clay, felt, and camera paper. Either the memories or the wine contributed to a warm inner glow I experienced and savored for nearly an hour. Thankfully, all I had left to do before morning was hang the children's annual Christmas ornaments on the tree.

I loved our Christmas tree. Years before, Heather had wished for a tree with complementary ornaments, garlands, and accessories. "Nothing matches, Mom. It's a jumble of old ornaments. Who'd want that?"

I wanted it. I always would. As she grew older, Heather changed her mind. She, too, savored the memories evoked by my old ornaments.

I hoped a little humor would dissipate the last of my moroseness, so I picked up *Paddy Clarke Ha Ha Ha* by Roddy Doyle. The book, a charming narration of a 1960s Irish childhood, with its innocent pleasures, surprises, and dares, was set against a backdrop of parental and Church authority.

My mood had improved by the time I heard, "We're back," from Bill. His shout instigated the dogs' barking. My reverie ended.

"How was the shopping?"

Bill kissed me on the cheek. "You didn't miss a thing, Pam. Crowds were so thick we could barely move." Eyeing me suspiciously, he asked, "How are you doing? Have you been crying?"

"I'm fine, really. I felt sorry for myself until I started reminiscing. I'm okay. Thanks."

"I'm afraid of losing you, Pam. I love you so much. I don't know what I'd do without you."

"You would be fine. You would probably marry some chick your daughter's age, with firm boobs and a nice butt, and you would forget about me in no time."

"I don't think so. Who would want an old fart like me?"

"I would," I said.

He kissed me. Jon walked into the room. "Gross! They're at it again. I'm going to get a complex, watching you paw each other like that. I'm going to need therapy." He tried to sound serious, but he burst out laughing.

I never asked Bill why it was okay for him to talk about losing me, but not okay for me to mention dying. I suppose I could have, but I appreciated the emotional support, so I didn't worry too much about the ground rules.

...

We were seated in church by a quarter to 11:00 for midnight Mass. Jon glanced at his watch every thirty seconds or so, sighing audibly. The boys whispered to each other, stifling snorts, grunts, and snickers. I felt obligated occasionally to give them a semi-serious, "Shh!" I didn't mean it, and they knew I didn't mean it, so the sniggering continued.

At exactly 11:30, the choir came to life, beginning with traditional hymns like *Silent Night*, *What Child is This*, and *O Holy Night*, and culminating with the popular songs of *Have Yourself A Merry Little Christmas*, *Jingle Bells*, and *White Christmas*. The boys looked bored. A few tunes from Bob Rivers, including *The Restroom Door Said, 'Gentlemen'* and *Wreck the Malls*, would have enlivened my bunch, but our church wasn't that progressive.

At midnight, the church bells chimed. As the two priests began Mass, I fondly remembered Christmases past—Christmases filled with hope and expectation. My favorite Christmas services involved parish children. One adventure-spirited group presented the story of Jesus' birth, complete with a heehawing donkey and an odoriferous sheep, which relieved itself on the way to the sanctuary. Despite Mary's efforts to comfort him, the baby Jesus' wailing drowned out the speeches of the diminutive actors. Amused, I imagined that scenario more closely represented the first Christmas, as opposed to the perfect Christmases celebrated in countless movies. It certainly mirrored life in my household, where I could only count on the fact that nothing ever went as planned.

Ringing bells snapped my return to the present. I uttered thanks for the years I had been given and added a hope I might have a few more Christmases to share with Bill and the children. The despondency felt earlier evaporated.

I sighed contentedly as we walked to our car after Mass. Peacefulness was supplanted by abject fear as I narrowly escaped injury by good Catholics negotiating their cars past obstacles in the parking lot—obstacles including churchgoers and other cars jockeying for a speedy exit. I slipped my arm through Bill's. He smiled, probably thinking me romantic. In truth, I decided that if my destiny dictated my demise at the hands of drivers obviously qualifying for the Indy 500, I was taking him with me.

...

Christmas morning. I woke to Heidi bathing my face with her sandpaper tongue.

"Need to go out, girl?" I squinted at the clock, trying to make out the time without benefit of glasses. "Wow! It's 7:00 a.m. Give me a second, girl." I slipped out of bed and pulled on a robe. It had been years since the kids nagged us awake by 0-dark-thirty to ravage presents. Trying to get my high school and college-aged kids up before noon had become the challenge.

I padded downstairs and prepared the dogs' breakfasts while they sniffed around outside. The scent of fresh coffee for Bill filled the kitchen as I whipped up our traditional Christmas breakfast of bacon and cheese croissants. They weren't exactly low in cholesterol, but we rarely gorged ourselves as we did on Christmas.

I savored a cup of cocoa while I read the morning paper. Afterwards, I called Mom, Dad, and my sister to wish them a *Merry Christmas* before the phone lines jammed for the better part of the day. I avoided mentioning my cancer. Nothing would change with waiting; I'd choose another day to ruin. It was 9:30 before anyone stirred upstairs.

After breakfast, we retired to the living room to open presents. Traditional Christmas carols had long been banned during the opening of gifts. Rob popped *Twisted Christmas* by Bob Rivers into the CD player. I was absolutely convinced Bill's classically oriented parents turned over in their graves every Christmas.

Now that the children were older, there were fewer presents to unwrap, although Bill insisted I still spoiled them—my prerogative. I'd put Bill in charge of buying the computer upgrades Heather wanted. I wouldn't have had a clue. I bought her two framed aerial photographs of the CU campus. A gold box tied with a pink bow held a gift certificate and a pair of thong, leopard-patterned, Victoria's Secret undies. Believe it or not, that gift was also from me.

"Nice gift, Mom. It isn't every girl who gets sexy underwear from her mother."

"You're probably right," I laughed. "I wanted to buy you a gift certificate, but the box looked bare. The undies were on sale."

"Glad to hear it."

Jon was in heaven over the computer upgrades Bill had picked up for him as well. The boxes for Heather and Jon contained different stuff for their computers, but the term upgrades was the only one I knew. Personally,

I didn't understand how anyone could get excited about pieces of machinery, but I listened attentively when the kids described how much more efficiently their computers would work when another piece was jury-rigged onto an existing machine that was state-of-the-art only six months before. I belonged to the era when a typewriter was the only piece of equipment necessary to create a semi-professional looking paper, albeit with crossed out words, type-overs, and erasures. If I had to change a paragraph, I re-typed the whole thing.

Being the attentive Mom I had always been, I pretended to understand Jon's chattering, but computer-ese was not a language I would ever master. It wasn't that I couldn't; I didn't want to understand it. I wanted to study nursing, medicine, languages, novelists, poets, and playwrights—not computer manuals, even if they did make them for *Complete Idiots*.

Computers weren't my only challenge. I'd also shown less than a stellar ability to choose gifts for my children. Gift certificates and cash had become my customary stand-bys. Although I promised myself I would always be tuned into whatever fads my kids loved, their passions often changed on a whim, and I had become too old, lazy, and frustrated to keep up.

I bought Jon a gift certificate to Crossroads Mall. He found it slipped between the folds of a dark blue pullover sweater.

"I never know what clothes to buy for you anymore, Jon. This way, you can pick out something you would really like."

"This is great, Mom. It'll be like having another Christmas." My kids were diplomatic if nothing else.

Rob asked for handcuffs. I assumed that was because he seriously considered embarking on a career in military law enforcement after high school. At least I hoped that was the case. Besides, most of his girlfriends were pretty stable. None of them would be into the whole S & M scene—at least I didn't think so. I found a pair of handcuffs I could live with: black, fuzzy Love Puffs at Spencer Gifts. They fit Hannah. Rob took a picture before she nibbled on them. He tore open the box holding his new stereo, but turned up his nose at the CD of Celtic music I'd wrapped.

"Ma! This is your kind of music," he whined.

"You might appreciate the lovely strains of *uilleann* pipes, *bodhráin*, tin whistles, and harps one of these days."

"Yeah, when pigs fly," he muttered under his breath.

I removed the CD from his hands. "Actually, this is mine. You and Jon may check out Camelot Music. Here's your gift certificate." Yeah, yeah—another gift certificate.

Hannah's patience with Rob's handcuffs came to an end. I burst out laughing.

"What?" Bill demanded.

"Those handcuffs on Hannah reminded me of Rob's plan to join the Army. Do you remember my telling you about that lunch at McDonald's on Ft. Bragg when Rob was three? He'd never seen anyone in an Army uniform, and there he was, surrounded by military men in camouflage fatigues. Right in the middle of the restaurant, he screamed, 'Mom, look! GI Joe, GI Joe!' I turned eight shades of crimson explaining you were in the Navy. The whole place cracked up."

I gently rebuked Bill for swinging his new golf clubs in the house, so he sheepishly sat down and stuffed his face with petit fours.

"Where's Mom's gift?" Heather cried out. "I don't see it."

"I've got it," Jon assured her.

Heather cleared her throat. The two boys stood behind her, grinning like they'd been caught ogling the centerfold of *Playboy*.

"Mom, we figured you could use extra protection right now," Heather said. "And we wanted you to know how much we love and appreciate you."

Jon handed me a small box. Inside was a cameo necklace—a guardian angel on a blue background. Sentimental fool that I was, I blubbered as Rob fastened the clasp around my neck.

"No tears today, Pam," Bill scolded. "This should be a happy day."

"I am happy, Bill. Really. And thanks to all of you." Hugs completed, I scooped up wrapping paper that had been shredded by the dogs. I thought they would have been munching on the rawhide bones I bought them, but just like toddlers, they were more enamored of the wrap than the gifts inside.

While I cleaned up the paper, Heidi chewed the felt antlers the children had placed on her head. Hannah and Holly had suffered years of indignities being dressed in pathetic outfits by the kids, so they quietly watched us, headgear intact.

The phone rang. It was Lisa, who worked as the referral clerk in our clinic. Lisa's job required endless forbearance, because she ran interference between insurance companies and us patient care providers. Regardless of the attitude of the individual on the other end of the phone, she remained soft-spoken and invariably pleasant.

"Morning, Pam. Finished opening gifts?"

"Just."

"What are your plans for the rest of your day?"

"We'll play some board games until the kids start arguing, and then we'll have the traditional stuff-and-groan dinner."

"No relatives this year?"

"No. Bill's sister was here last year, and my sister hasn't made the arduous trek to Colorado yet. This year it's a quiet family Christmas."

"Small family, I take it."

"It is. I have one sister, and Bill has a sister and brother. We have the only children on both sides. I've occasionally hinted to Heather that she might as well elope when she finds the right fellow. There won't be anyone on our side of the church."

"You've lots of friends..."

"I have, and I'm grateful—especially now."

"How are you holding up?"

"As well as I can. I know that sounds cryptic, but I have such extreme highs and lows, I'm beginning to wonder if I'm manic-depressive."

"I'm sure what you're feeling is normal, Pam."

"I feel anything but normal, Lisa. I have this insidious disease making its home in my body, and I'm not happy at all. I'm really not."

"I'm so sorry."

"Ah, don't be. I'll get through this. I abhor feeling sorry for myself. When I get past this, life will be great."

"You'll get through it; you've got fantastic friends to help you."

"Yeah, and they sound pretty humble today. Merry Christmas, Lisa."

"Merry Christmas, my friend. I have an ulterior motive for calling today."

"Do you now? And what might that be?"

"Would you have lunch with me at Karen's tomorrow? I'd love to steal a couple hours of your time."

"That would be lovely. Shall I pick you up?"

"I've a few errands to run. How about if we meet at the restaurant at noon?"

"Great. I'll see you then. And thanks, Lisa."

"No problem. Talk to you tomorrow."

Off the phone, I asked, "Who's for a board game?"

Rob, ever the comedian, asked, "Did you say b-o-r-e-d game?"

Chapter 7 - December 26th

Karen's Country Kitchen graced the corner of Main and Pine Streets in downtown Louisville. Built circa 1894, the structure was consecutively a drugstore, bank, post office, and law office, before being transformed into a gift shop and bakery in 1974. Over the years, starving patrons encouraged Karen's menu expansion to three meals a day.

The Country Kitchen's light lavender and purple trimmed façade, with maroon fabric awnings, appealed to locals and visitors alike. Inside, the walls were lined with shelves and cupboards full of enticing cookies, candies, and gifts. The motif reminded me of an old-fashioned general store, chock-full of items. A multi-tiered, refrigerated glass case stood to the right of the reception counter. It housed some of the most delicious cakes I'd ever savored—and I had the figure to prove it.

Instead of my usual drooling, I hurried past the cakes in search of Lisa. As usual, the restaurant was packed. I looked through several rooms in search of my friend. I was late and feeling guilty about it.

"Pam!" Lisa called, seeing me frantically scan tables.

"Sorry," I gasped breathlessly. "I decided to walk and realized I was going to be late, so I ran the last ten minutes. I hope I don't offend anyone."

"We'll know you have if people move their tables away from us. I'll be glad to give you a ride home if you leave the window down."

"Thanks for the self-esteem boost, Lisa. It's great having loyal friends around when your deodorant fails."

"How did your Christmas end?"

"I couldn't sleep."

"Worried about the cancer?"

"No, actually I'm still concerned about Andrew."

"That little fellow with pneumonia?"

"Yes."

"He must be doing better, Pam. Wasn't he discharged from the hospital?"

"He was, but that doesn't keep me from worrying. And his parents are back from vacation. I'm sure his recovery is downhill from here."

"That was really nice of you, by the way."

"What was?"

"Spending the night in the hospital with him while his parents were away."

"I enjoyed it. His poor grandfather couldn't care for Andrew's sisters and stay in the hospital at the same time. And two-year-olds don't cope in the hospital without parents very well. I was the logical choice; at least Andrew knew me from the clinic. Mom and Dad flew home as soon as Grandpa called them...He does that every year, you know."

"Who does what, Pam?"

"Andrew's grandfather is spending his retirement years circulating from one child to the other, giving them yearly ten-day breaks to travel, while he watches the grandkids."

"What a guy!"

"He was great."

"So, you couldn't sleep last night."

"Not a wink. I got up and walked on my treadmill for an hour."

"Did you watch a movie while you walked?"

"I did. It helped me keep my mind off Andrew.

"And did your movie feature Gabriel Byrne, perhaps?"

I laughed. "It did. I watched *Hello Again*. Gabriel Byrne plays a caring emergency room doctor. It's nice to see that once in a while. A lot of the ER docs I have worked with suffered serious delusions of grandeur."

"As opposed to the majority of actors, of course."

"You're probably right, but I've read that Gabriel Byrne is a kind and generous man who has charitable interests that go miles beyond his bank account. He's not the only one, of course. Actors like Liam Neeson, Harrison Ford, Tom Hanks, Paul Newman, and Mel Gibson have great personalities and big hearts as well. Their movies dress up my drab little life."

"And your source for all this useless information, Pam?"

"Mostly *People* magazine—my one vice in life."

"Your only one?"

"The only one I'm willing to tell you about, Lisa."

I marveled at the uniqueness of the restaurant for probably the fiftieth time. An enterprising architect expanded the restaurant by incorporating the beauty parlor next door into its renovations. Instead of destroying outer walls to create one large room, he maintained the adjacent external walls, complete with windows, and placed flooring over the dirt walkway that ran between the buildings. Skylights dotted the ceiling over the walkway. As a result, one could enjoy a short stroll between curtained windows walking from the front of the restaurant to more seating in the back.

At one point in its transformation from law office to celebrated restaurant, a designer ingeniously used weathered doors as backrests for booths and fashioned discarded window frames into tabletops. Fabric-covered lampshades and lace curtains transformed each room into a turn-of-the-century parlor. The alluring effect was polished by the use of a mélange of fabrics, wall coverings, and various furniture styles. Paintings for sale by local artists graced the walls.

"Ready to order, ladies?" inquired our waitress.

"I'll have a Cobb salad and iced tea," Lisa replied.

"Make that two. It'll be an extra half hour on the treadmill tonight," I sighed.

"What are you doing with your free time these days, Pam?"

"I'm reading a lot. I love reading mysteries, but I've become fascin-ated with Irish history."

"Hmm. Could your interest in Irish history have anything to do with a dark-haired, brooding Irish actor?"

"Why does everyone call Gabriel Byrne brooding, Lisa? I've read he's a very funny guy. Although I enjoy many of his movies, I've liked Irish actors for a long time. When I was a kid, I loved movies starring Richard Harris and Peter O'Toole. *Lawrence of Arabia* is one of my favorite films. The first time I saw that great epic, I watched it at a drive-in movie, trying to appreciate the heat and aridity of the Nefud Desert while our windshield wipers ineffectively swiped at raindrops the size of golf balls."

"Most people who go to drive-ins aren't there for the movies, Pam."

"True, but I went with my mother and sister."

"Oh. That's an entirely different story. Personally, I think that Liam Neeson is pretty easy on the eyes."

"I can't disagree with that, Lisa. Actually, I'll admit I did begin read-ing about Ireland because I wanted to understand the culture from which my favorite actors came. I recently finished O'Toole's two-volume autobio-graphy: *Loitering with Intent—the Child* and *Loitering with Intent—the Apprentice...*"

"Could I borrow Peter O'Toole's biography from you, Pam?"

"Of course." I paused. "I've lost my train of thought, dog gone it."

"Sorry, Pam. My fault. You were talking about wanting to understand the Irish culture."

"Right. Thanks. The Irish are amazing. They struggled for nearly eight hundred years to rid themselves of oppressive rule. Millions suffered horrendous deaths. Many leaders of their revolutions were teachers, farmers, poets, and writers. When they were beaten down, they rebelled again. Now I'm fighting for my life. I'm going to fight this cancer as though it was the cancer that infested the Irish Isle. And like they did, I'm going to win."

"Methinks there is passion in the woman."

"There is. If it takes passion to conquer this, you're looking at a very passionate woman. Do you think I'm crazy being interested in a culture so different from my own?"

"No. I'm fascinated by English history."

"We learned a great deal about British history in school, but that translated into history that affected the English. I didn't learn anything useful about the Irish—or the Scots and Welsh for that matter."

"We didn't fight the Irish for independence, did we, Pam?"

"No, they had their own struggles with the English."

"They did."

"I've another project besides reading about the Irish people, Lisa."

"What might that be?"

"I'm writing a book."

"A book is very ambitious."

"It is, but I want to write about my struggle with cancer. If for no other reason, the kids might enjoy learning how their mother's pathetic mind works."

"You might scare them if they get to know you too well."

"I can't deny it. I read somewhere that journaling during illness can be mentally and emotionally beneficial."

"That's true, Pam. I've heard it's very cathartic."

"That sounds like a laxative, Lisa. I will write a book that will purge me of my despair." We laughed.

When our salads arrived, Lisa said, "How about filling me in on what you're facing the next few months. After lunch we can take the dogs for a walk, if you'd like."

...

Lisa drove me home to collect my dogs. We packed Holly, Hannah, and Heidi into my kid-trashed vehicle after I scooped up and discarded

Burger King wrappers and soggy soda cups. I futilely brushed dog hair off Lisa's seat. The hairs stuck straight up in the upholstery, and nothing but picking them out one at a time was effective. Lisa politely laughed at my heartfelt effort. I hoped she'd ignore the dog drool and nose prints on her window.

She *was* sitting in the dogs' seat after all. And just like my three kids, the dogs fought over who got to sit in the front seat next to Mom, the remainder being relegated to the back seat to pant noisily in my ear. My admonitions that they "be nice to each other, girls" usually got the same response it received from the kids—total disregard.

We headed out Highway 93 to Dowdy Draw Park. Boulder County provided a number of parks where animals were permitted off leashes to romp and chase indigenous wildlife. During the summer, the scents of pungent cow pies proved challenging to breathing, but at this time of the year, the concerns were more banal, and less olfactory, involving how much grime the dogs could amass gamboling through muddy fields.

Lisa and I walked briskly through the first of a series of gated fences that provided sanctuary for domestic livestock. The dogs surged ahead in quest of rabbits and rodents, but hopefully not skunks. Watching them frolic, I let my lazy mind drift back to Bill's naval tour on Mare Island, California, when the submarine he had commanded was overhauled. Mare Island was overrun with skunks, a fact that Holly relished and I dreaded on a weekly basis. At least that often, I'd hear a bark, followed by a squeal, and the unmistakably pungent odor of skunk. After slinking back to the house, Holly would roll on the ground in a vain attempt to rid her body of the overwhelming stench. This weekly routine reduced me to bathing the suffering, and did I mention stupid, canine in tomato juice to dissipate the odor. As I laboriously heaved the stinking dog into the downstairs bathtub, I unleashed diatribes that resonated through the house. Those words probably still hung loosely in the atmosphere over the Golden Gate Bridge, ready to haunt me when I stood before St. Peter.

"How dumb can one dog be?" I would demand. Hey, I wasn't going to leash the dog to do her business and risk *my* coming face to face with a cute, but smelly little black animal with a white streak running down its back. Even Penny, our older golden retriever, kept her distance after one encounter with a skunk. But Holly never learned. Of course, my ire was not lessened by the fact that Holly shook frequently during her bath, showering both walls and me with tomato juice. Holly's blond hair remained a delicate shade of pink for days after each incident, and she kept a bit of distance between herself and me for about twenty-four hours after her baths as well.

"You seem lost in thought, Pam," Lisa remarked.

"Sorry. I was thinking of all the times Holly was sprayed with eau de skunk when we lived in California. Man, did that stink. She never learned. She's the dumbest dog I've ever known, but she has a sweet disposition. Long ago, I decided God gave her two hearts and no brain."

We walked in silence for several minutes.

"It's beautiful out here, Pam."

"It is, Lisa. It's gorgeous. I can almost touch the mountains. Bill, the kids, and I have lived near many mountains over the past twenty years, but none have touched me the way the Flatirons do. Looking at those mountains on a clear day, with clouds hovering around their peaks, gives me an incredible sense of peace. I could happily roam these fields forever."

"Pam, if you would take your head out of the clouds and observe the many fragrant piles of cow droppings at your feet, you would remember this is not the best place to be in the middle of summer. But otherwise, it isn't bad." She looked around. "Where's Heidi? I only see Holly and Hannah."

My stomach knotted. I took in the whole pasture, easily locating Holly and Hannah. I finally spotted Heidi several hundred feet ahead, racing hell-bent through a muddy field.

"Dear Lord, she's black!" I hollered. "My blond cocker is black."

"I know who's having a bath tonight, Pam. In fact, judging by the color of the other two blondes running through the fields, you are going to be a busy woman this evening. It's a good thing you brought towels for the back seat."

"Too bad I don't have Bill's jeep instead of my car," I grumbled. "I don't mind getting his car filthy."

"I'll gamble he doesn't share that sentiment."

"You'd be right. He loves that car. Jeeps are supposed to be rugged, off-road vehicles, but that car has more bells and whistles than you can imagine."

We walked to the end of the path overlooking the valley. The base of the Flatirons bordered the far side.

"Lisa, there's got to be a way down this cliff to reach that field and cross to the base of the mountains—without breaking our necks. Look at that farm in the valley. What a view! I'd give a lot to own that property."

"I can see it all now, Pam. The nurse practitioner in the field, standing under a cow ready to deliver a calf. Then, a rush to slop the hogs and plant the corn before dawn breaks. All of that would be followed by a hearty breakfast for your brood before dashing off to tend the horses."

"Okay, so maybe I'm not destined to be a farmer's wife. But it sure would be terrific to have a place with a view like this. Maybe when I win the lotto..."

"You have a better chance of being struck by lightning," Lisa retorted, "which may be a strong possibility considering those black clouds rolling in. I think we should collect the dogs and get out of here," she screamed as the skies loosed a torrential downpour.

Chapter 8 - December 29th

After tormenting myself vacillating between options, I scheduled my second surgery right before New Year's Day. Ironically, I faced the same decisions as several of my patients. As had been true of them, my mind muddled with unwelcome emotions. Fears crept through the trenches of my mind like insidious creeper vines, intent on strangling every bit of rational thought I possessed. Now I understood the conflicts patients experienced, weighing options. I'd held them as they cried, confused, begging me to make decisions for them. Of course, I couldn't. I encouraged sharing fears with loved ones, who would provide emotional support. They understood they could call me with questions, and they frequently did, but the final decisions were theirs.

Weathering the consequences of those decisions occasionally brought pain. Theda Marshall, a sweet-natured, plump lady of forty-nine, suffered through the anguish of three benign biopsies before hearing the dreaded diagnosis of cancer. Her two sisters, her mother, and two aunts had waged battles with breast cancer. Two of them endured recurrence in the other breast. Fear of death pervaded Theda's waking thoughts, and frequent nightmares tortured her sleep.

"I've decided a double mastectomy is my only hope of peace, Pam. My surgeon says breast reconstruction at the time of surgery is an option, and my insurance company will pay for it. Is that right?"

"That's right, Theda."

The exam room door banged open. Theda's husband stormed into the room.

"That's it?" he screamed. "You're going to do it? You're going to have them both lopped off?"

Tearfully, she nodded.

"Fine!" he raged, spittle punctuating each word. "Then I'm leaving you! Deal with your decision the best you can! I want nothing to do with a deformed freak!" He charged from the room. Tears spilled down Theda's cheeks. Her body convulsed with loud, wracking sobs.

I wanted to tear that bastard apart. My mouth gaped and I stared at the open door. I refused to believe the scene had happened. No man could be such an ass. I stood, determined to chase after the worm and loose my contempt upon him, but some power greater than mine forced me to absorb the anguish of the woman beside me. I gathered her in my arms as best I could and let her cry until she was spent.

Later, I called that miserable excuse for a man and pummeled him with my wrath. He slammed the phone down before I finished, but I felt better.

Theda stayed with her mother through her ordeal. A year later, she purchased a lovely two-bedroom condo. She reveled in her job at a local hospice. She often volunteered to share the appearance of her reconstructed breasts with women contemplating the procedure.

"Aren't they lovely?" she'd beam. "Fifty-one and perky breasts. I love 'em. They feel so natural—go ahead. Sneak a little squeeze." Theda loved herself. Her dirt bag husband left the area and, hopefully, was rotting in hell.

I decided against a mastectomy, and it had nothing to do with Bill's attitude. Or maybe it had everything to do with it. He told me he loved me for myself, and my breasts, or lack of them, had nothing to do with it. That meant so much to me. Forget the housework he'd never done. With that one comment, he'd wiped out every bad mark on his eternal chalkboard. My bad marks, I imagined, were still pending.

I gambled that survival odds for infiltrating ductal cancer were almost equivalent for simple lumpectomy versus complete breast removal "with appropriate post-surgical treatments", of course. Bill appreciated my difficult choice. Knowing my love of humor, he made light of the situation one evening.

"I checked my health insurance policy today," he said. "There's a dismemberment clause that will give us money if you lose one of a pair of essential organs. Breasts aren't considered essential, so there's no monetary advantage in having a mastectomy versus a lumpectomy."

"Not essential," I quipped. "Obviously a policy written by a person unconcerned with self-esteem issues. However, since this breast has been part of my life for forty-five years, I've decided to keep it. I'm having a lumpectomy."

My greatest fear was loss of consciousness from general anesthesia required for the coming surgery. A local anesthetic could not deaden the axillary tissue well enough to permit painless harvesting of lymph nodes. Harvesting. It put me in mind of a shaft of wheat, blowing in the wind.

Pathology analysis of the nodes would provide a sense of the cancer's possible spread. At the follow-up appointment after my first surgery, Dr.

Jones indicated he would enlarge my previous incision and excise further tissue.

"Pam, according to the pathology report, the tissue margins weren't clear. That means there is still malignant tissue I can remove."

I listened to him, but sometime during the conversation, depression invaded my thoughts. The silent prayer begging for divine intervention would not be granted—there would be no miraculous revision of my cancer diagnosis.

Because my surgery was scheduled for 7:00 p.m., Dr. Jones decided I should spend the night on the oncology ward after leaving recovery. Dressing for the hospital, I reflected on the cancer's increasing impact on my family and me. Over the past couple of weeks, I'd reveled in joyous memories, like reading to my children when they were young. I'd often found myself re-reading favorite books *ad nauseum*. After a while, they *read* those same books to me, making up the most delightful stories to accompany the pictures.

"And then the doggies ate the flowers, and then the mommy said, 'No, doggies, don't eat my flowers', and then the mommy took the doggies to McDonald's, and ..."

We were very fortunate Bill was stationed in San Diego during those early years, since I worked nights to meet our mortgage payments. My boss, Ginger, understood a sleepless day followed each night at work, since I'd be caring for three rug rats. She rarely scheduled me to work two nights in a row. My zombie mind failed to put more than a couple of words together until blissful sleep refreshed me twenty-four hours later.

A college student slept over when I worked, and I always arrived home in time to help the children play with their breakfast. I don't believe I fed our golden retriever, Tigger, while the children were small. She remained devotedly at their sides, keeping the floor cleaned of dropped food particles and gently lapping up proffered food from their tiny hands.

The kids didn't care if I could put two thoughts together after being up all night. They demanded hugs, fun, and stories—in that order. I bought family passes to Sea World and the San Diego Zoo/Wild Animal Park. We frequently—read several times a week—ventured to the realm of wild and woolly animals. We spent days hiking and foraging through parks and children's museums. We rarely knew from one month to the next whether Bill would be home or not, so the five of us took advantage of the magic of Disneyland and Knott's Berry Farm in Anaheim when we could.

Occasionally, Ellen, a dear neighbor, took the children overnight. Bill and I spent a few blessed hours without the pitter-patter of little feet running down the hall and tiny hands banging on the locked bedroom door.

"Whatcha doing, Mommy?"

Those wonderful nights, we dropped off the kids at Ellen's and ate at a forbidden restaurant (meaning anywhere it took longer than three minutes to cook an entire meal). We spent the rest of the night, well, not sleeping much. I always reciprocated, hoping our friends had as much fun as we did.

I never regretted a moment I spent with my children—at least that's what I told myself in later years. Selective memory was wonderful. I'd conveniently forgotten the tons of diapers, illnesses, sibling fights, school projects, and overwhelming fatigue.

I'm grateful the children always shared life-shattering concerns. Over the years, we talked about every imaginable subject. In fact, it wasn't uncommon for them to drag friends home to ask my advice on humiliating topics. I encouraged their friends to talk with their parents, but for some, dropping an embarrassing situation in the lap of a stranger prevented personal mortification.

My kids never experienced reticence about asking *me* embarrassing questions. Maybe that's because I was a nurse practitioner in addition to being Mom, and as such I had access to top-secret information—in their minds, anyway. I'll admit questions they asked were sometimes difficult to answer *because* they were my children. However, I believed it was better for them to learn facts than obtain misinformation from peers with big imaginations or a bigger Internet. And, I rationalized, I could interject a little morality into most lectures. I tried to be subtle. If I was not particularly successful at the subtle part, the kids rolled their eyes, which was my cue to back off.

I'd noticed however, that since before Christmas, everyone was treading lightly around the unexploded time bomb—me. They surreptitiously watched me, waiting for the "Thar she blows!" which never came. Unusual for them, they weren't asking questions. I didn't feel like volunteering much information, so I didn't. They were worried and I should have deflected their fears, but I couldn't, feeling so full of fear myself. I wanted to appear strong for them, although a bowl of Jell-O pretty much summed up my courage most days. Like a child choosing between cleaning his room and eating a bowl of Brussels sprouts, I vacillated between wanting to crawl into a shell and spilling out every anxiety. I longed to go to bed and wake hours later, finding the nightmare had vanished. I still felt sorry for myself frequently, and although I understood the mood swings, I found them difficult to accept.

I hoped that once cancer treatments were over, I would enjoy life again and not become preoccupied with the disease. Just as cancer could literally eat my tissue, mentally it could nibble away at my soul, depriving me, and anyone around me, of joy. I didn't want that to happen. I prayed for guidance.

Bill, too, weathered my emotional roller coaster in unexpected ways. He became more solicitous, encouraging me to discuss my feelings, although talk of death was still banned by me. Our lovemaking changed, too, if you don't mind my mentioning that. After the passion was spent, instead of rolling over and going to sleep following a quick peck on the cheek (which had always been his custom), he held me in his arms until I separated from him. I was grateful. Since Christmas, he had taken on many household chores without being asked. He still refused to believe his helping around the house turned me on.

"Right!" he'd said, mocking me. "Well, it doesn't turn me on." Since it never took much to turn him on, it didn't matter.

I thought that my diagnosis of cancer and fears related to the future would lead to a decreased desire for sex, but it hadn't. In fact, Bill's willingness to help around the house, and my desperate need to feel attractive despite the changes occurring within, had culminated in my turning to him more frequently—a need he was more than happy to satisfy.

I sighed. Reminiscing allowed me to avoid the issue at hand, but the challenge of my next surgery still stared me in the face. I grabbed the overnight bag I had haphazardly prepared for the hospital and walked downstairs. Bill finished an early dinner and put my bag in the car. Driving to the hospital, we conversed little, but he held my hand, occasionally giving it an encouraging squeeze.

"No matter what the outcome, Pam, I'll be there for you, and we'll get through this together."

Reassurance was all I needed.

...

"Mrs. Stockho?" A young nurse glanced around the waiting room. These days, they were all young. Another squeeze from Bill and the two of us walked through the now familiar doors to the day surgery suite. Rapidly undressing in my tiny cubicle before I became frostbitten, I placed all my clothing, except my socks and underwear, in a plastic bag. This time, I added my glasses. The world was a swirling blur of abstract designs and colors.

"This is when a seeing eye dog would be welcome," I blurted out as Bill peeked around the corner. "Remind me to increase my donations to *Guiding Eyes for the Blind*. Uh, that is you, isn't it Bill? Things are pretty fuzzy over here on this gurney, and I'm not getting out from under these warm blankets to make sure you aren't a masher."

"It is I. Decent?"

"Always decent for you, dear."

Amy, my nurse, pulled back the curtain. "Ready for your IV? I'm going to start warm saline before Dr. Thornton comes in to talk to you. She's the anesthesiologist. She will discuss putting you to sleep for the surgery."

Amy found a vein in my right hand, but moving the needle slightly caused it to infiltrate. A bruise spread over the back of my hand.

"Oops, sorry about that. I'll look for a vein on the left side."

I tried to stop her diplomatically. "Uh, my surgery will be on my left breast and axilla. Do you think it might be a problem starting the IV over there?"

"It could be. Maybe your husband can apply pressure to your hand while I look for a vein higher up on the right. Sorry. There's going to be quite a bruise."

"Don't worry about it. I've missed a few veins in my career."

"Are you a nurse?"

"Yes, but I haven't worked in a hospital for a long time. I especially miss the emergency room."

"The ER can be exciting, Mrs. Stockho. I worked there myself for about fifteen years before burning out. I couldn't take the stress anymore. This job is satisfying and a lot easier to leave at the end of my shift. I can finally go home and sleep at night without worrying about patients."

"I know what you mean, Amy."

A woman stuck her head into the room—I couldn't describe her, because I'd surrendered my glasses and was blind as a bat. Thankfully, the soft-spoken physician refrained from sticking her face in mine, but that also meant she remained a blur.

"You about finished, Amy?" she asked. "There isn't enough room for another body in this room."

"IV's in, doctor. She's all yours."

After reviewing my past medical history and allergies, Dr. Thornton listened to my lungs and heart. "According to records, you refused sedation during your last procedure, but this time, I'm going to give you Inapsine. By the time you hit the operating room door, you'll be out for the procedure. The anesthetic I'll give to you today is short acting, so you should wake up from your surgery quickly, with little residual grogginess."

An OR nurse appeared. "We're ready for her, doctor."

"All right, I'm pushing the Inapsine." I was asleep before I could decide if the gurney wheels were out of alignment.

...

"Pam, wake up." My brain was fuzzy. "Pam? Can you hear me?" The voice became clearer. I moaned as I opened my eyes.

"Are you in pain?" my recovery room nurse asked. I focused on her face, but wasn't sure if the drugs or my lack of eyewear blurred her. I squinted, but it didn't help at all.

Was she smiling? I probably was a sorry sight right then. "My name is Gwen," she said. "After I get a set of vital signs, I'll give you Demerol for the pain and Phenergan to prevent nausea. Your husband is waiting in your room; we'll have you upstairs in a jiffy."

...

Gwen and an oncology floor nurse, Sarah, helped me scoot from the gurney to the bed. My head needed bolting; it lolled from side to side. Whoopee! Fuzzy brain, fuzzy brain. Oops! My gown wasn't pulled down well. No worries! They'd seen it all before, hadn't they? Yee hah!

"I have warm blankets for you, Pam. Just ease over slowly."

Are you talking to me? What are you saying? Scoot my butt over? Grin. You keep on talking, but the words reach my brain in slow motion. What did I miss? Scoot, scoot. Stuck to the sheets. Yo! Hold that gurney closer to the bed. My rear's falling through. Scoot, scoot.

"You're almost on the bed, Pam. A little farther."

Scoot, scoot. Singsong in my brain. Look at all these tubes. I look like a machine. Pain in my chest, but the drugs make me not care so much, la la. Scoot, scoot.

"Great. That'll do it, Pam. I've got to check the drains and your dressing, get a set of vital signs, and then you can rest."

Sarah placed my call bell within reach and explained the operation of the bed and television. Uh huh! Whatever you're saying. Yup! Head lolling a bit. Shaking the cobwebs from my brain. Fuzzy, fuzzy. Sarah checked the bulky dressings over my breast and axillary wounds. She pinned the drains to my gown so they wouldn't pull on my skin. Sweet of her. She was talking again, but what was she saying?

"...and the drains prevent blood from pooling under your skin because of the more extensive incisions made during this surgery. They will be removed when you return for your follow-up appointment at the surgeon's office."

I flashed Bill what I thought was an acceptable smile, but he shook his head. "Pam, what did they give you? You look like your mind's having a great time."

Wider grin. Slurred speech, but just a little. "Why don't you go home, Bill?" I asked with difficulty. My mouth was filled with marbles. And dry, very dry. "Just gonna sleep, sleep deep."

"That sounds like a plan," he agreed.

Sarah tucked warm blankets around my shivering body. "This is a hospital, Pam. No sleep for you. Short periods of rest are all you'll get. I'll be taking vital signs every fifteen minutes for an hour and then every hour times four. By the way, if you have to use the bathroom, buzz me. I don't want you falling on the floor in the middle of the night. Dr. Jones will see you in the morning to discharge you. You can plan on your husband taking you home after breakfast, about 8:00 a.m. Dr. Jones makes his rounds early, although he may stop in to see you this evening."

Bill leaned over the railing and kissed me goodnight. Our lips almost made contact.

After he left, Sarah turned out the light, and I rested for a few minutes. I drifted in and out of sleep. By the time she returned to take another set of vital signs, my brain had cleared. She checked my temperature, blood pressure, and pulse, and then pulled a chair up to the side of my bed.

"You may not remember me, Pam. I came to see you for back pain about a year ago. I had a kidney infection. I was in agony. The aching and fever almost did me in. You were so compassionate—I'll never forget that. I've told everyone about you. Several of my friends have been to see you. You cared, and that meant so much to me. I'm sorry this happened to you."

I was touched. Tears sprang from my eyes. I'm sure the narcotic had a bit to do with my labile emotions, but nevertheless... "I'm going to be fine, Sarah. Whatever happens, I'll be okay. And I appreciate the referrals."

Sarah hugged me.

"Watch that left side, young lady," I begged.

Dr. Jones strolled in. "I wanted to make sure you were tucked in and comfortable." He checked my dressings and drains.

"My boobs haven't had this much attention in a long time," I said.

"I'll have to speak to your husband about that."

"Other than him, I meant. Speaking of spouses, shouldn't you be on your way to see yours? It's almost 10:30."

"If I'm home before eleven, she figures something's wrong. I'll see you in the morning to discharge you."

After he left, I remained awake for a long time. I made out a few water-stained areas on the ceiling, thanks to the nightlight Sarah left on. At least I thought they were water stains. I squinted, but I couldn't be sure. Where were my glasses?

The pain in my left breast and under my left arm was a constant reminder of the cancer that, hopefully, had been mostly removed. Undoubtedly, cancer cells had navigated my blood stream to seed else-where. Tears welled up. Feeling sorry for myself had become exceedingly easy. I didn't want to resort to becoming a mountainous glob of self-pity, because it wouldn't accomplish anything. But lying there, alone in the shad-shadows afforded by one single bulb, I felt incapable of dredging up any other emotion. I gave myself up to weeping.

Chapter 9 - December 31st

Two days after my second surgery, the drains were pulled in Dr. Jones' office. After examining my breast and axilla, he pronounced the sites healing well, with only moderate induration and swelling. He checked the strips of adhesive covering my incision sites.

"Pam, leave the steri-strips in place until they fall off, probably in a week or so. They'll give support to those suture lines so, hopefully, your scar will be less noticeable."

Sure—as if the world would have an opportunity to gaze upon those scars, noticeable or not, I thought wryly.

"You may bathe or shower," Dr. Jones continued. "Call the office if you notice signs of infection like redness, swelling, fever, or increased pain. I'll call you as soon as I receive the final pathology report." He answered my questions and patted my arm, smiling benignly. Most of the questions I'd written down were for the oncologist.

"I know this is difficult for you, Pam." He couldn't know how I felt, but he was sympathetic and compassionate, and I was grateful.

"Please call the office if you have further questions. Most patients with breast cancer are anxious to begin treatments. Ask your primary care doctor to initiate a referral for the oncologist, so you can make an appointment to see him in about two weeks. The tissue must start healing before the next treatment phase begins." I nodded silently and left his office, fearing the next phase, but anticipating another positive step to eradicate the disease.

•••

Pain prevented me from raising my left arm higher than my shoulder, so I'd been wearing button-down shirts and cardigan sweaters. Changing my bra remained a major undertaking, but it gave extra support to my agonizingly aching breast. I chose to avoid narcotics to control pain except to sleep. They dulled the pain, but left my brain incapable of any rational thought.

I readied myself for a shower, gasping at the horrific pain as I removed my bra. I quickly cupped my breast with my right hand. The pain lessened. I wildly wondered how I could shower and wash my hair with one hand. I had not realized how much my bra and the dressings prevented pulling on my suture lines. I wept as the weight of my breast tugged at my healing tissues.

I turned to face the mirror, gazing for the first time at Dr. Jones' handiwork. The red incision line on my breast was approximately four inches long. Mildly indurated tissue below the incision line pulled the nipple up slightly. My breast looked perkier, but now it was a little off-line compared to the right.

The observation reminded me of CPR courses I'd taught. Placement of the hands for cardiac compressions approximated the nipple line on a male. Because women's nipple lines changed with time—being more fluid in position, so to speak, students were taught to place hands two finger-widths above the xiphoid process, an anatomical part not challenged by age, breast-feeding, or gravity. The bits of flotsam, which drifted through my consciousness, were ridiculous.

I examined the cavity left after the cancer's removal. It wasn't as large as I thought it would be, but I wouldn't be able to fully evaluate it until the swelling decreased. Most of the breast tissue above my nipple was hard and painful. Raising my arm as much as I could, I examined the incision line under my arm. Approximately three inches in length, it felt tender and swollen. Two stab wounds, one under my axilla and one just lateral to the breast incision, were all that remained of the drains. I attempted to raise my arm above my shoulder and cried out in pain. I wondered if I would ever feel normal again; on the other hand, many of my friends would challenge I'd never been normal in the first place.

I turned on the water and stepped into the shower. Although left-handed, the only way I could manage washing my hair and body was to hold my left arm close to my body, cupping my sore breast in that hand, while I used my right arm to lather and rinse. It was extremely awkward. I dropped the soap at least a half dozen times and blindly reached for it as water and my hair kept me from seeing clearly—as clearly as I could see at the best of times without eyeglasses. I slipped on the bar of soap twice. After that, I leaned against the shower wall and cried. Heidi whimpered and clawed at the shower door. I opened the door, and despite being lathered with soap, I reached over and gave her a pat.

"I'm okay, girl," I soothed. "I'm fine." Heidi cocked her head, looking up at the pathetic woman she called Mom. I attempted a smile, which Heidi probably couldn't see through the hair plastered to my face.

Finishing my shower, I stepped out and felt around for a towel. I brushed my soaked hair from my eyes, shooting water across the room. It took nearly twenty-five minutes to shower and towel off, more than three times longer than usual. I didn't feel clean; soap still clung to strands of hair, but I wasn't about to get back into the shower to rinse it out.

Another downpour of tears escaped as I stupidly grabbed for a towel with my left hand to wrap around my hair. Pain shot through my breast like a dagger. I almost dropped to my knees. I had no idea there would be so much pain. The incisions were not more than a few inches in length, for goodness sakes. But the pain was real and the nightmare inescapable. Dear God, am I going to die? I wept uncontrollably.

After several minutes of feeling sorry for myself, I pragmatically decided that standing around in a damp towel wouldn't help me accomplish anything. Getting dressed remained a huge challenge. If the situation had not been so pitiful, I could have made a fortune selling a video of my getting dressed to some comedy show. I was cold, a perpetual problem for me, and I was tired of wearing cardigans. I eased a bulky sweatshirt over a turtleneck. Too late, I noticed the sweatshirt was stained. I usually crossed my arms over my head to pull off sweatshirts, but that was not an option now. It took several frustrating minutes to ease my right arm out of the sleeve and gently pull the sweatshirt over my head. I lost it, screaming at myself in the mirror—a big help surely.

"You are pathetic, woman!" I flung the sweatshirt on the floor. Tears flowed again. I had constructed quite an emotional roller coaster for myself: way up, way down, way down, down, down.

I awkwardly pulled back my shoulder length hair with a large barrette. "Don't I look gorgeous?" I facetiously asked the face in the mirror. And didn't I feel it, too? I thought.

I sat on the edge of the bed. I hated my weakness. Hopefully, time would banish my despondency. And time I had. Recovery from surgery would necessitate an additional week at home. I wondered what project might elevate my mood.

I willed myself to entertain bright thoughts. My happiest thoughts, of course, embraced memories shared with three children, three dogs, and one husband. Those reminiscences were forever captured on bits of photographic paper haphazardly stored in boxes in the basement. Some were more than five years old.

I had separated older pictures into four albums (for each of the kids and myself) the year Heather and I spent in Virginia Beach, but I'd sorted none since. Organizing the products of my over-active camera into more albums was a dream for the future. I glanced at Heidi, who sat statue-like in front of me, her head cocked uncertainly.

"Well, girl, it looks like Father Time has gotten my attention. I'd better get my lazy butt in gear and tackle those future plans." Then, I'd clean closets and cabinets before undertaking a bit of writing. Anxious to start, I headed to the basement.

After Heather moved into the apartment near school, I redecorated her basement bedroom, creating not only a guestroom, but also a respite from Bill's frequent window-rattling snoring recitals. I'd always wanted a room that engendered a sense of tranquility. Over twenty-five years, I'd collected many unusual frames, and they surrounded over eighty of my favorite family photos. I displayed them on built-in shelves and on every available inch of a desk and dresser.

I framed twenty-two of my Catherine Grunewald prints. The intricate details of whimsically animated folk art prints, capturing pastoral scenes, heavenly bodies, and earthly creatures, always cheered me. Catherine proved to be every bit as ethereal and blithesome as her winsome pieces; I was privileged to have spoken with her twice in Williamsburg, Virginia. We exchanged a few notes over the years. Catherine's exuberance and kindness filtered through to me in my sadness. I stood before her print, *Let It Rain*—four smiling angels sharing a day amid sheep and planted fields. Let it rain, indeed, I thought, my sad mood dissipating as the angels lifted my weary spirit. I'm going to beat this!

My home away from home in the basement served as a library of sorts. I had collected many American and Irish books on history, politics, and folklore. An oak bookcase housed tomes by poets and novelists, as well as picture books depicting the magnificent glories of the States' and Eire's past and present. Many spilled haphazardly onto the floor, and hundreds of books I'd read through the years lurked behind the closed door of my storage room.

Bill swore I bought too many books, but I didn't believe I would ever have too many. Besides, I told him, books multiplied at will. Many jumped right into my arms as I strolled through Barnes and Nobles, Borders, or Waldenbooks. Although I often entered shops intent on purchasing only one title, I never left with less than half a dozen. I could have developed worse faults than a love of reading, in my humble opinion. Thank God for libraries, or my literary bills would have bankrupted Bill long ago.

Since getting sick, however, I'd read less and watched movies more. Between work and thinking about cancer, my poor brain remained under siege nearly twenty-four hours a day—even my dreams were nightmares I'd not experienced since childhood. Movies permitted mindless entertainment, and for a time, I embraced that.

...

Books and movies were not on my mind as I lugged boxes of photos from the storage room. Family pictures were scattered all over the guest-room bed when the front door slammed. I glanced up at the clock—I'd been working on my sorting project for nearly three hours.

"Mom, I'm home for lunch," Rob called out. "Where are you?"

"In the guest bedroom downstairs," I hollered up to him.

"Whatcha doing?" he demanded, his eyes drinking in the chaos I had wrought. He stared at me. "I haven't seen you this happy in weeks."

"I'm organizing family pictures. It's a total pain, but as you can tell from my face, a total pleasure as well. I wish I had labeled each bundle with dates when they were developed. I'm trying to remember where and when I took all these snapshots. I've got lists all over the bed."

"You have your work cut out for you, Mom. Are you at a point where you can stop? I thought it might be nice to have lunch with a nice, old broad today. What do you think? How about Wendy's—my treat."

"If you're buying, I'm all for it. Thanks. You're a great kid. Have I ever mentioned that?"

"Yeah. I think you've mentioned it once or twice."

I stood up to hug him. "Ma! The hair! Don't mess up the hair! I've got English this afternoon."

"English?"

"Yeah, English. I'm trying to make a good impression on one of the girls in my class."

"Forgive me for mussing up even one hair follicle. I'll settle for a free lunch instead of a hug." I left my pile of photos and strode upstairs with my boy, intent on creating new memories.

Chapter 10

After our lovely lunch, I returned to organizing pictures until Bill came home. He found me, much the same way Rob had, by hollering until I answered. Before dinner, Bill gathered the clan. Issues had arisen.

"It's time to verbalize feelings about what's happening to Mom—about what's happening to all of us."

Oh, oh, I thought. I hated being the center of attention.

"Are you up for discussing this, Mom?" Heather asked.

"I'm not sure, but I suppose this is as good a time as any. We're walking around on eggshells. Everyone's afraid to say anything."

"How do you tell your mother you're afraid she may die?" Jon blurted out.

Blunt, very blunt, but surely a sentiment on everyone's mind. "God willing, I'll be around for a while, gang, but one never knows with breast cancer. Surgeries and treatments often kill enough cells so the body can fight the rest, but sometimes, despite best efforts, standard treatments aren't enough. Even if I die as a result of this, it isn't going to be for a while. I have plenty of time to make your lives miserable. If I'm granted a long life, I'll thumb my nose at everybody."

"Since you're willing to discuss this, I would like to say this has made me very angry," Heather said. "I felt selfish saying anything since you're going through so much, Mom."

"Let me say something, if I may," Bill replied. "We may not be physically involved, but we're definitely emotionally involved. Whatever you feel is okay. None of us should keep this bottled up. That includes your mother." He faced me. "Pam, you've been especially quiet and preoccupied these past few weeks. You need us as much as we need you. I know sharing feelings makes you uncomfortable, but please don't shut us out."

My man was a marvel! I swallowed hard. "I'll try to be more candid about how I feel, but that's not easy. Please understand that when I appear introspective, I'm trying to cope—trying to keep from falling apart. You've got to admit I've been blubbering a lot lately."

"It's okay, honey," Bill assured me. "We're here for you, whatever you need. We love you." He put his arm around me and gave me a peck on the cheek. Oh, God, the tears started again. Rob grabbed tissues from the bathroom.

I dried my eyes and blew my nose. "Heather, you wanted to share some thoughts," I said.

"I do, Mom. Like I said, I'm angry. First of all, on a personal note, I'm angry this may happen to me."

"About eighty percent of breast cancer is random and not hereditary, Heather," I told her. "Genetic testing may indicate whether or not you have a predisposition to breast cancer, but the results may be used against you by insurance companies when they assign health benefits."

"No, I don't want to know at this point. I'm just mad cancer showed up in our family. I mean, why you?"

"The question should probably be, 'Why not me?' No guarantees come with life, honey. Frankly, it amazes me that human bodies function as well as they do. We take so much for granted. We expect these frail shells to protect us from disease and injury no matter how we treat them. I wonder how, in such an uncertain, polluted world, these bodies protect who we are so well." It was certainly easier to say that than feel it. I didn't want to be sick.

I continued. "Heather, I will, unnecessarily, point out that you are female. That makes you susceptible to breast cancer, whether or not I had ever developed it. However, research and treatments keep making huge strides forward. Every year the prognosis for a long and healthy life increases."

"That won't help you," Heather murmured.

"Of course it will, darling. My chances of beating breast cancer are much better than even a few years ago. I'm trying to have an optimistic outlook, most of the time anyway. Once I recover from surgery and get through my treatments, I'll try to put this behind me and enjoy life once again."

"You're not the only one hoping for a bright future," Rob said. "Have you seen the tabloids lately? The world is supposed to end in the next year or two."

"A little pessimistic, aren't you?" I asked. He was sneaking dog biscuits to Hannah, whom I'd recently nicknamed Chubs, under the table. "Hopefully, we'll all live a very long time, Rob. The world will not end in the next year or two. I forbid it. Actually, I don't believe God would do that to me—as if it really makes a difference how I fare in the great scheme of things." I sighed. I wanted to lighten up the discussion a little. "This year, for me, will not be one I remember with great fondness. I am looking forward to next year and will not be happy at all if the world comes to an end. Besides, I want to visit Ireland and zoom around town in a classic 1970s Mercedes 450 SL, and I refuse to die before your father grants those two wishes. And that's final."

"How can you joke about this, Mom?" Jon demanded. "God, if I had to go through what you're facing, I'd really be depressed." He scratched Heidi's back, so she rolled over, granting him the honor of massaging her tummy. The look in her eyes convinced me she was in doggy heaven.

"I wallow enough in despair, believe me," I said. "But that doesn't change the situation. I'm allowing myself a bit of anger, sorrow, and grief. This is an emotional process, like any other. Hopefully, my emotions will stabilize over the next several months. I refuse to let my ravaged body dictate my life as long as I feel relatively healthy."

Bill growled. "I'd like to ravage your body."

I laughed. "Down, boy! Later."

Jon rolled his eyes. "That's disgusting, you guys."

"What?" I exclaimed. "I'll remind you of that little comment when you reach your mid-forties. I guarantee you will be a long way from rolling over and playing dead when you get into bed with your wife at night."

"Gross!" But there was a twinkle in his eye. Heather remained quiet.

"Heather, did you want to say something else?"

"Mom, I'm really upset about cancer treatments. You mentioned you are probably facing chemotherapy. I wish you could avoid that."

"Thanks," I said quietly. "Except for this inconvenient little problem, I'm pretty healthy. We'll deal with chemotherapy one day at a time. If I'm really sick, I know I can count on all of you to pamper me, bring me meals in bed, and take my dogs for walks. Right?"

The kids avoided my eyes.

"You can probably count on their help as much as usual," Bill said. "But I'll be there for you, sweetie. I'll take care of the meals when you don't feel up to it. We can do a new five-meal plan: McDonald's, Domino's pizza, Kentucky Fried Chicken, Tulien's Chinese food, and Olive Garden take-out. We'll rotate those five meals until you're back on your feet. How does that sound, kids?"

"Great!"

I shot Bill a dirty look. "We'll all be as fat as pigs. And where's the good stuff, like fruits and broccoli?"

"Broccoli, yuck," Bill said. "We can get veggies on pizza, and some Chinese dishes comes with veggies, including broccoli. And the Olive Garden has great salads."

"As if any of you would order salad if you weren't forced. Just because former President Bush hates broccoli doesn't mean you can get away with it. Think of all the vitamins and minerals in every little floret."

"Yuck," Bill said again.

Rob chimed in with, "Don't sweat it, Mom. Dad's got the meals all covered. You feel free to be as sick as you want."

"Thanks a heap. Why do I get the feeling you're not taking this meal discussion seriously?"

"Because we're not," Bill laughed. "And it's certainly great to see five smiling faces for a change. We haven't had a lot of that these past weeks."

"Jon, you haven't said much," I coaxed. "Do you want to share anything else?"

"Not much. It's been hard thinking about returning to school. I'm worried about you getting around, wondering if you'll need things done. Stuff like that."

"You concentrate on school. Your father will be around. What do you think I married the old fart for? I won't be an invalid. I'll only be out of commission a couple of days each cycle. As I said, I will live it up. I'll lay in bed with my handy dandy puke bucket and watch *Usual Suspects* and *Miller's Crossing* until I can't see straight."

"Remind me not to interrupt you when you're either throwing up or watching your favorite movies. Both those activities make me sick," Jon kidded.

"You're just jealous," I teased.

"Of what, puking or watching the same movies a dozen times? Seriously, and I'm changing the subject here before I get any more nauseated, is there any book that might help me understand what you're going through?"

"The one I recommend to patients is *Dr. Susan Love's Breast Book*. The information is excellent. It's upstairs by my bed. Feel free to borrow it for a couple of weeks."

"Say," Jon interjected, "I just had a thought. Talk about ironic. How come Mom, who eats well and exercises, got cancer, and Dad, who smokes, sits on his butt watching television, and has been around nuclear reactors and nuclear waste products for more than a quarter of a century, is healthy as a horse?"

"You want to take that question, Bill?" I asked.

"I have better genes than your mother," he said, semi-seriously. "Besides, even though I've been around hazardous environments, there are tons of safety precautions. I haven't been exposed to any significant amounts of radiation—certainly not much more than all of you are exposed to, walking around in the sunlight."

"You mean you don't glow in the dark, Dad?" Heather asked. "I'm disappointed."

"Don't worry. Your mom and I have never had any trouble finding each other in the dark."

"Whoa," Jon remarked, holding his arms up in the form of an X. "Not again. We are quickly getting into the realm of 'this is more information than your children need'."

"I don't mind Mom and Dad talking about sex," Rob interjected.

"Yeah, well I think old folks ought to show a bit of restraint in that department," Jonathan interjected.

"Old?" I countered. "I'll have you know I'm not past my prime yet."

"Yeah, right," Jon snickered.

"Do you hear how your son talks to his mother?" I demanded of Bill.

"No fair talking about the old bag like that," Bill rebutted.

"Something tells me Dad is not going to be getting any tonight," Rob joked.

"Dad had better watch his step," I agreed.

"Dad," Heather asked, "has Mom's cancer made you think about your smoking? I wish you'd quit."

"Going through a difficult trial like your mom's cancer is not the time to give up a bad habit like smoking. I'll try in a few months, though. I promise."

"The man has promised before," I replied. "He won't give it up until he's ready. You think I can be a grump? Man, you don't want to be around your father when he gives up the weed. At least he doesn't smoke around us. I can't ask for more than that."

"Young lady, how are you going to visit Ireland and enter all those nasty, smoke-filled pubs if you can't tolerate a little cigarette smoke?" Bill teased.

"Young, am I now? Are you trying to get into my good graces? Well, you're still on probation after that last cheap shot. As for the pubs in Ireland, I'll just hold my breath."

"That I'd love to see," my husband shot back, playfully giving me a squeeze.

"Hold it, Bill. What did you just say? Something about a trip to Ireland? Are you serious?"

"I've been thinking about it for a while. After your treatments, let's do it."

"Yes!" I kissed him.

"I think Mom's forgiven Dad for his tasteless remarks," Rob decided. "Maybe he'll get lucky tonight after all."

"Let's not go there again, ok, Rob?" Jon pleaded.

"Is there any further discussion on this subject tonight?" I asked. "Any more comments directed at your poor, pathetic mother?"

The only sound came from Holly. "Woof!"

"Guess someone wants dinner." Two of the three dogs jumped into the air.

"They aren't the only ones," Jon added. "I'm starving."

"She'll probably make us eat broccoli after all that," Bill grumbled.

"As a matter of fact…." I laughed, heading out to the kitchen.

...

That night, Bill held me. "You're beautiful," he whispered.

"You're horny," I replied.

"That, too. But I won't touch you until you're ready. You can't be too comfortable," he added, aware of my squirming.

"I hurt no matter how I lie here," I sobbed. "Bill, I'm scared."

"So am I, sweetheart. But we're going to get through this together, I promise. Say, were you serious about that old Mercedes?"

"I was. I want an old convertible to tool around in before I kick the bucket. I shouldn't say old. Maybe classic. That sounds right."

"Well, if you want one before you die, I'd better get started on a hunting expedition right away." A look of horror crossed his face. "I didn't mean that the way it sounded. You're going to live a long time. I just want you to have everything you want."

"I know that, Bill. You're sweet. It's great you would even think about buying me an old car that will probably need lots of money poured into it."

"I don't mind pouring money into an old, er, classic broad like you, do I?" he asked.

In response, he got a hug. He kissed me and turned off the light.

I listened to his steady breathing, which quickly gave way to snoring. I tossed and turned for an hour. Earplugs were not helping. I rose, put on a robe and opened the door. Heidi was quickly on my heels. The devoted dog, I thought, reaching down to pet her.

"Well, girl, I can't sleep, so if you would like to come downstairs and spend a couple of hours watching a movie with me, I'll provide a dog treat."

I poured a small glass of wine and popped *Point of No Return* into the VCR. I might not be able to sleep, but a movie would keep me from feeling sorry for myself for a couple of hours.

Chapter 11 - January 15th, 1999

Despite the decorator's skillful utilization of color to foster feelings of peace, I experienced renewed tension entering the waiting room of the Rocky Mountain Cancer Center. Muted colors of purple, gray, and aqua dressed the walls, furniture, and carpeting. Abstract paintings complemented the color scheme. Splashes of color were haphazardly brushed onto canvas and metal. I thought wryly that my poor brain had been suffering a similar chaotic jumble since I'd first heard my diagnosis.

Much of one wall housed a tropical fish tank. The vibrantly colored fish darted from one end to the other. I felt as trapped as they were. I shivered. I could not run away from cancer. I had to deal with it, but I felt very ambivalent. On one hand, I wanted to start treatments as quickly as possible. On the other hand, the beginning of treatments would mean I had finalized decisions regarding the course my therapy would take, and I had no crystal ball to indicate the path that might provide the best chance for survival. Silence permeated the room. The walls closed in around me. My chest felt heavy and I hyperventilated. Bill noticed and he hugged me.

After signing in at the desk and handing over my insurance co-pay, I sank into an overstuffed love seat and watched a steady stream of older, mainly hairless people, shuffle in and out of the office. I daydreamed they were all young again, with happy faces and great expectations for the future. I forced myself from my self-imposed reality retreat by studying those around me. An older gentleman with steel-gray hair guided a woman to a seat. I shrunk deeper into my chair as I watched the woman's pallid, drawn face. She looked apprehensive. She appeared tiny, almost lost inside a billowing purple caftan. She frequently adjusted a turban on her bald scalp. The woman shot me a hesitant smile as she sat down.

Interminably long minutes passed by. A young lady entered the office and scanned the silent waiting room. Settling on the woman dressed in purple, the young lady strode in her direction.

"Sorry I'm late, Mom and Dad," the young woman sighed. "Has Mom's blood been drawn?"

"We've just been here a few minutes. She hasn't been called yet," her father replied a little louder than I thought necessary. I felt cranky. I gave him the benefit of the doubt, thinking he might be hard of hearing. "Mom's been slow getting going today."

A door at the far end of the office opened, and a smiling, blonde-haired woman, probably in her mid-twenties, looked around. Her eyes rested on the lady in purple.

"Mrs. Abraham. Are you ready for blood work before we start your chemotherapy today?"

Mr. Abraham watched his wife shuffle toward the lab. He shifted his position to sit closer to his daughter. His voice boomed. "It's great having you to talk to while Mom gets her treatment, Tammy. It's been a long haul. You never know how she's going to feel. Mom's been puking her guts out on and off the last couple of weeks. I don't know how much more of this chemotherapy she can take. And, of course, you never know if they've got it all. The damn microscopic cells can be growing anywhere. Just when you think you're making progress and that you're going to whip this thing, you find out the cancer's spread God knows where. This is really wearing me out."

Shut up! I thought angrily. How dare he bellow out comments like that when I was sitting in this jail, anticipating being called to hear my sentence? I was on death row, hoping for a reprieve. I knew what he said was true, but I could bear no pessimism now, before I'd even met with the oncologist. I almost rose to ask the receptionist to tell Mr. Abraham to pipe down, but instead I withdrew into a protective shell. I felt Bill's reassuring hand on my knee, but it gave me no comfort.

Tears trickled down my cheeks and I wiped them away with the back of my hand. The stabbing pains in my left breast and under my arm continued to remind me of surgery. Would the pain ever fade? Would I ever stop feeling sorry for myself?

"Mrs. Stockho?" a pleasant voice called out from a door behind my left shoulder. "I'm Barbara Evans, the office manager. We need a few insurance forms filled out before your consultation with the doctor."

Following silently behind her like a whipped dog, I was overcome with a desperate desire to scream. This is not happening! I am healthy! This is a horrible mistake! Not me, please dear God, not me!

The corridor ended at the door to a large conference room. Large sliding glass doors, leading to a balcony outside, framed one side of the room. Black mesh covered every inch from the roof to the balcony.

"Did you put up the netting so people can't jump off the balcony when they hear their prognoses?" I interjected lightheartedly, trying to improve my dark mood.

81

"No," Ms. Evans replied, obviously missing my poor attempt at humor. "It keeps the birds out." She gave me a warm smile. "Here are the forms you need to fill out. I'll be back in a few minutes in case you need help. Dr. Sitarik will be in shortly.

After Ms. Evans left, I walked to the windows. I didn't feel like filling out forms. Hoping to mentally erase the reason for my being there—fat chance—I peered out the windows. The peaks of the Flatirons rose in the distance. For the briefest moment, I experienced tranquility. I drank in their beauty before reluctantly turning from them. As I walked back to the table, I perused the numerous texts and periodicals lining the bookshelves that covered an entire wall. Every one of them was devoted to cancers and their treatments. So much cancer, I mused.

Bill, God bless him, was dutifully filling out insurance forms and questionnaires. He was almost finished when Dr. Sitarik walked in. I noticed the doctor's smile first. I saw confidence and kindness in that smile. His black hair framed a handsome face and sparkling brown eyes that were full of encouragement: I care about you. We are in this together. For the first time since I'd heard the word cancer, hope surged through me. His grasp was strong and reassuring.

"Good morning, Mr. and Mrs. Stockho. I'm Mark Sitarik."

"Please call me Pam."

"Fine," he said. "Pam, before I examine you, I'd like to review the pathology and blood work reports. I know you're a nurse practitioner, but because this information can be intimidating when you're the patient and not the provider, I'm going to review this in layman's terms. Your husband will probably appreciate that." Bill nodded. "By the way, Dr. Bachelder called. I'll be answering to her if I don't take good care of you. Please stop me if you have questions."

He flipped through the chart. "The CEA blood test indicates whether the tumor has spread to other parts of the body. We oncologists don't usually order this test when a patient presents with a small tumor, because the test isn't sensitive enough to locate small groups of scattered cells. We do order it when we suspect a tumor has spread extensively. Since your surgeon ordered it, I'll tell you that the result was less than 0.05. Normal is anywhere from zero to three. So that's good, although, as I indicated, that doesn't necessarily mean body organs are free of migrating cancer cells. Research into breast cancer is increasing, thanks to improved public awareness, and new tests are being developed which are more sensitive.

"Your tumor was relatively small, 1.5 cm or about three-quarters of an inch. The prognosis generally improves if the tumor is small, but there are no absolutes when discussing breast cancer. This is where I interject an admonition to patients. Women with breast cancer tend to berate them-elves for not finding the tumors earlier, for not having had a mammogram sooner, or not having done their breast exams often enough. It's important to do breast exams and have mammograms, but neither is a guarantee that tumors will be found at an early stage. Much depends on the type of tumor, its location in the breast, whether calcifications show up on a mammogram, etc. Please don't waste precious energy torturing yourself. Sometimes a tumor isn't found until it is already extensively metastasized, or spread, to other parts of the body, and sometimes that's the earliest it could have been found with our current technology. I know you may think it's easy for me, a man, to say don't worry about what you could have done differently, but, on the other hand, about two percent of breast cancers occur in males."

"I know," I agreed quietly. "I teach male patients to do breast and testicular exams when they come in for physicals. Occasionally, they laugh, but it's just as important for them as it is for women. I recently sent a thirty-six year old male to Dr. Jones for a breast lumpectomy. I was describing what a suspicious mass feels like when I felt a firm, immovable, one-centimeter lump in his left breast. Hopefully, it won't be cancerous."

"I wish all practitioners would do the same," Dr. Sitarik remarked. "Thankfully, preventive health care is gaining importance. Even though your cancer is beyond the preventive stage, your self-checks helped pick up the tumor fairly early. It distresses me when a woman relies solely on a mammogram to detect cancer. It's a great tool, but it doesn't always pick up early tumors.

"As you probably know, Pam, there are two predominant types of breast cancers. About four-fifths of these cancers begin in the breast ducts and the majority of the remaining tumors start in the breast lobules. There are a few other miscellaneous breast tumors, but they make up a very small percentage. Your tumor is an infiltrating ductal carcinoma, which means it has progressed beyond the duct in which it started. It's the most common type of breast cancer."

"I've heard it called a 'garden variety' type of tumor."

"That's an interesting way to put it," Dr. Sitarik mused. "Ductal cancers have a slightly decreased chance of occurring in the other breast compared to lobular cancers, and ductal cancers are also a little easier to detect. Lobular cancers send out projections into the tissue without causing much inflammation, so they're harder to feel, and the surgeon may have difficulty removing the bulk of the tumor. Otherwise, the prognosis for both cancers is about the same. The good news for you is that although one tumor margin showed active cancer growth after the first surgery, the margin was clear after the second surgery. So it appears Dr. Jones removed the bulk of the tumor successfully.

"The lymph nodes removed from your axilla were negative for cancer, and that's great, but that also can't guarantee cancer hasn't spread elsewhere. Tumors encourage the growth of new blood vessels, and this new blood supply transports cancer cells all over the body. Thankfully, we have a wonderful immune system whose white cells attack cancer cells and, hopefully, kill most of them before they infiltrate other organs. You have to remember, though, that by the time you feel a lump, the cancer has been growing for several years."

"Why does it take so long for tumors to get large enough to feel?" Bill asked.

"Good question," Dr. Sitarik remarked. "Cancer cells divide and double about every hundred days. In aggressive cancers, a larger proportion of cells divide at any given time compared with less aggressive cancers. A tumor measuring about a half inch in diameter, and that's on the small side of being palpable, contains about one hundred billion cells. That's a lot of cell division and takes several years. Does that help, Bill?"

Bill nodded.

"Regardless of what you and I decide to do, Pam and Bill, we're not going to know for a very long time whether or not we 'got it all'. It may be ten to fifteen or more years before a tumor is large enough to be detected elsewhere. I'm not trying to be pessimistic here, but you have to understand what you're facing. This information impacts your decisions regarding treatment. Although most of the tumor has been removed, there are probably tumor cells at the site of excision and there are likely to be cells that have traveled through the blood stream to other organs. Unfortunately, we don't yet have the technology to determine which tumors are genetically more likely to metastasize throughout the body. The technology is coming, but it will still be a number of years. Do you have questions at this point?"

"No," I said. Exhaustion set in. "Some of this I know. I'm trying to concentrate on what you're telling me."

"Assimilating all I've said can be difficult at the first visit. I'm glad you brought your husband."

"Like I know what you're talking about," Bill muttered under his breath.

Dr. Sitarik chuckled. "Please continue to ask questions as they arise, Bill, and call the office if you have questions." He waited a couple of minutes before proceeding.

"There is good news here, Pam. Fewer than five percent of the cells in your tumor were actively dividing. That means this is a less aggressive, slower growing tumor.

"Biomarkers were also examined, specifically those receptors related to estrogen and progesterone. Both were positive. That's good, because we can give medication that will decrease breast tissue sensitivity to female hormones. The prognosis, therefore, with positive markers is somewhat better."

"Doesn't that also mean I'm going to have a miserable menopause, because I won't be able to take hormone replacement?"

"It's possible, Pam. And chemotherapy, which I recommend, can force you into an early menopause. You may stop having periods and may have hot flashes. After chemotherapy is completed, your periods may or may not return."

"So, after chemotherapy everything may be back on track? I may not go through menopause for a few years?"

"Recovery of your ovaries often depends on how close to menopause you are when you begin chemotherapy. And since your tumor is responsive to estrogen, I'm going to recommend you start tamoxifen as soon as your primary treatments are completed."

"Which means what exactly?" I asked.

"Tamoxifen, which I encourage you take for five years, may contribute to menopausal symptoms. It blocks estrogen receptors found in the breast, although it *acts* like estrogen in some other organs like the bones and uterus. For example, the risk of osteoporosis in women with a family history doesn't appear to increase while one is on tamoxifen. There are some side effects other than hot flashes and mood swings though, such as depression, eye problems, and a slight increase in endometrial cancer. The latter has mainly been observed in postmenopausal women, and the percentage is small. Women who have a strong family history of breast cancer may decrease their risk with prophylactic tamoxifen."

"This isn't the best news I've ever heard, Dr. Sitarik."

"It isn't, but there are a few non-hormone medications that can help with menopausal symptoms. For instance, women have found that a small dose of the anti-depressant Effexor is helpful in combating both hot flashes and the depression that occasionally occurs with tamoxifen. Let me know if any menopausal symptoms become a bother for you."

"I will. Thanks."

"You're welcome, Pam. We're nearly done." He waited until I nodded before continuing. "Since we've delved into the realm of treatments, let's talk about them. I recommend you begin chemotherapy within the next few weeks. Five weeks of radiation will follow. Then I recommend tamoxifen for five years."

I swallowed hard but said nothing.

"Chemotherapy destroys cancer cells that have infiltrated other organs. Although there is no guarantee chemotherapy will destroy all the abnormal cells, it is hoped the number will be decreased enough to allow your immune system to kill off the rest."

I sighed. "Is this the same immune system that is depleted to possibly critically low levels by chemotherapy?"

"It is. But it should bounce back somewhat between treatments."

"Should—I like that positive thinking, doc," I said.

He flashed me a smile. "Your chemotherapy will consist of six, three-week cycles. The drugs I recommend are cyclophosphamide, methotrexate, and 5-fluorouracil. This treatment regimen, known as CMF, is less toxic than others, although there are still many potential side effects. A treatment nurse will review drug information. The more common side effects include hair thinning, mouth ulcers, and mild fevers. Your platelet and white blood cell count will decrease, making you more susceptible to bleeding and infection. Fatigue may be significant and cumulative over several months."

"This doesn't sound like much fun."

"No, I can't say these will be the best months of your life. But the alternative…"

"Is much more unpleasant," I agreed. "I'm afraid, Dr. Sitarik."

"Of course you are, Pam, but please remember we're here to help you get through this. We'll be with you every step of the way."

"I appreciate that, Dr. Sitarik."

"Do you have any more questions, Pam?"

"Are there as many side effects with radiation?"

"No. It's a relatively safe procedure these days. Radiation is concentrated in the breast from which the tumor is removed, hopefully destroying microscopic cells left after surgery. Since cells may have migrated to other parts of the breast, the entire breast is irradiated. For five weeks, five days a week, you'll receive treatments at the radiation therapy center. Treatments take only a few minutes. Hopefully, after these treatments, you'll never need others. However, I will point out that if the cancer recurs, radiation will not be utilized again. Normal cells previously exposed to radiation are less capable of repair if irradiated again." He paused. "Do you have other concerns?"

"Dr. Sitarik, how do you feel about alternative treatments, like dietary changes, acupuncture, homeopathy, herbs, or biofeedback?"

"Deciding on a course of treatment is highly individual, Pam. Personally, I want controlled studies before embracing alternative therapies. At this time, I can't recommend any in place of traditional medicine. As adjuncts to chemotherapy and radiation, however, many patients have found changes in diet, regular meditation, acupuncture, and herbal supplements helpful. Herbs that decrease menopausal symptoms *may* stimulate estrogen receptors in the breast. I've found no scientific studies examining that particular aspect of peri-menopausal herbal preparations, so I would advise you to avoid them. Some herbs and acupuncture help with unpleasant side effects of chemotherapy, such as nausea and anorexia. This is Boulder; we have a number of excellent herbalists and specialists in Chinese medicine. Additionally, many patients find relaxation tapes and biofeedback helpful to reduce anxiety. I can recommend someone if you like."

"Thanks, but Dr. Hibbard's wife, Chris, is a specialist in biofeedback. She's leant me some relaxation tapes. She'll help me if I need her. May I ask if you have many patients who opt for the herbal, acupuncture, or organic food route in lieu of chemotherapy and radiation?"

"Honestly, no. I've a few, and I support a woman's choice. I make sure she understands the risks inherent in abandoning traditional medicine, but the final choice is hers."

"The choices are difficult."

"They are, Pam. Treatment of breast cancer may radically change in the next few years, but at this point, I believe the regimen I've proposed is best for you. I admit chemotherapy and radiation have limitations—not all women are helped significantly. Some cancers have already spread extensively by the time they're diagnosed, which offers little hope with even our best cancer-fighting tools. But mental outlook plays a vital role in one's prognosis; I firmly believe that. Feel free to examine various therapies and incorporate them into your treatment plan. Is there anything else you would like to discuss today?"

"Yes. Will I be able to work? My bosses are very understanding, but they have to make plans."

"Most women continue working at least part time. Fatigue may limit your hours. With your depleted immune system, you will need to avoid anyone who is sick."

"Doctor Sitarik, most of the patients I care for have colds, pneumonia, diarrhea, vomiting, and other contagious illnesses."

"Oh. That changes things. Generally speaking, the white cell count reaches its nadir between days ten and fourteen of the three-week cycle. As long as your count isn't dangerously low and rebounds as expected, you should be able to work the first and third weeks of each cycle, staying away from the office the second week."

"Okay, Dr. Sitarik. That can be arranged."

"After the first treatment, we'll check your cell counts on days ten and twenty-one. For this first cycle, however, I want you out of work the entire three weeks to see how you respond to treatment. I'm assuming you agree with me on the regimen we'll take."

I nodded. "I'm not thrilled about subjecting myself to chemotherapy and radiation, but I believe the regimen you propose will give me the best chance of fighting this. I'm placing myself in your hands. Last week I was perusing Dr. Love's book. She mentioned that if a simple lumpectomy is done, the risk for recurrence in that same area of the breast approaches thirty-seven percent. That's not a percentage I want to worry about. I wish there were proven alternatives. I'm reading about therapies utilizing an individual's own white cells to decrease the incidence of side effects. I'll be so grateful when patients don't have to face the toxic medications we do now. Ah well. I think I'm about questioned out. Bill, do you have any more questions?"

He shook his head.

"We'll talk to your nurse if we come up with any earth-shattering concerns. When do you want me to start chemotherapy?"

"Let's plan on the end of next week. That will be just over three weeks since your last surgery. It will also give your clinic time to replace you during the first treatment cycle. I think you'll do fine, Pam. So, if neither of you has further questions, I'll have my nurse take you to an examination room. I'll be there shortly."

Thanks to Dr. Sitarik's kindness and patience, decisions were made. I'll admit that my gut still wrenched every time I thought about the poisons I would allow in my body, but I trusted him and believed he was arming me with the best artillery to win the battle.

Chapter 12 - January 18th, 1999

"Spill the beans, Pam," Lisa demanded three days later, as she made lunch for the two of us in her kitchen. "I want to know every sordid detail of your oncology appointment."

I lusted after Lisa's house. The place was spotless. She had no children to leave telltale signs of every daily activity (unless, like so many of us, she considered her pets—two cats—her children). The sink was free of dishes. No food remnants remained on the table. No jackets graced chairs. No shoes or backpacks impeded walking up stairs. Lisa and her husband lived in a tidy home free of dog drool and dog hair.

I treasured her friendship. She was intelligent, hard working, and perpetually happy. She helped sanity reign in our clinic, and that was no small feat.

"Pam?"

Suddenly aware I'd been daydreaming, I returned my attention to Lisa and her look of anticipation. I hadn't answered her challenge regarding my oncology appointment. While she tossed a salad, I reviewed that momentous occasion. Despite having agreed with Dr. Sitarik's therapeutic regimen, her question elicited renewed anxiety.

"I have concerns about the proposed treatments, Lisa, but if I refuse chemo and radiation and the cancer advances, I'll drive myself crazy wondering if it might have been different had I followed Dr. Sitarik's advice. However, there are times I can't believe I'm considering subjecting myself to toxic chemicals and X-rays that both have the small, but real, potential of causing cancer themselves."

"You still have significant reservations about your treatment plan, don't you?"

"I do. But I'm putting my faith in my doctor. I want to beat the odds, and he's convinced this is the way for me to do it. Honestly, at this point I just want to get treatments started. Once I've had the first one, I won't vacillate back and forth. It will be a *fait accompli*, so to speak. I want to move on. I want to feel healthy again. Do you think that will ever happen? How can I put cancer out of my mind when there will always be the nagging possibility it may recur?"

"I don't know how you'll accomplish that, Pam, but I know you. You are very strong-willed. You won't allow illness to defeat you without a fight."

"You're right, Lisa. I have patients to care for and books to write."

"How goes the writing?"

"Pretty well. I'm writing my story as I go along, so I won't forget details. The funny thing is, the book is evolving in third person. Ann Kennedy has cancer. I still can't say, 'I have cancer'."

"I can understand that, Pam. Where did the name Ann Kennedy come from?"

"It's a nice Irish-sounding name, but I can't give you more reason than that. It popped into my head. Since I'm on a fiction roll, I'm going to have Ann Kennedy write a letter to her favorite actor, known in the novel as Kevin Scanlon."

"Interesting. And in this highly fictionalized account of your, excuse me, Ann's breast cancer, does Kevin Scanlon write her back?"

"He does. Not only that, but they meet."

"Ah. And do they have a torrid love affair?"

"No. Ann's married. I can't make her *that* different from me. After all, I'm a short, calorie-challenged, forty-five year old mother, not a twenty-something model.

"Ann Kennedy could be a twenty-something model."

"Nope, she and I are kindred spirits. Ann and Kevin become friends and that's it. He helps her through her cancer treatments."

"That sounds lovely. Totally romanticized rubbish, but lovely. There's no way a book like that would sell, but it's lovely."

"Why wouldn't it sell?"

"People want passion and sex, or sweaty sex without passion, not the ramblings of a married forty-five year old with cancer."

I pouted. "I have sex."

"You're married. It doesn't count. No one wants to read about married sex. It's too plebeian."

"Says you!"

"I do. So who is helping *you* cope with your cancer?"

"You, for one. And my family."

"Me? I don't know anything about cancer. What am I doing?"

"You're here for me. I've got my oncologist and colleagues to help me with cancer information. I just want to surround myself with people who care about me. I don't need anything more."

"You know you can count on me."

"I do. I'm very lucky. I've gotten loads of calls and letters from my sister, parents, and friends."

"On that tender note, I will tell you that lunch is served."

Lisa was a fabulous cook, although I believed anyone who enjoyed cooking was a fabulous cook. It was ironic that I despised preparing meals, despite my having done so for a hungry family for over twenty years.

"You know," Lisa once remarked, "if I had to dream up tantalizing entrees for three kids who complain about food that doesn't taste like pizza or hamburgers, I'd hate cooking too. Is Bill picky?"

"No, he'll eat anything except Brussels sprouts and broccoli, and even then I can occasionally get away with it if I disguise the offending vegetable in sauce. This looks great, Lisa. You make cooking look easy," I whined.

"I don't spend one day each weekend slaving over a hot stove whipping up the following week's menu. Unlike you, I don't get home from catering to cranky patients until 6:30 or 7:00 p.m. If I knew I *had* to shop every Saturday and cook most of every Sunday, I'd hate it too. I have the luxury of cooking when I feel like it and eating out when I feel like it. Steve cooks too. Now stop whining or I'll cripple you."

I shut my mouth and stuffed my face with salad.

"I've always wanted to write a book, Pam, but just the thought of organizing enough material to make a book is daunting. At least typing on a computer makes things easier. Right?"

"I won't dignify that with an answer," I pouted. Actually, I didn't want her to know I hadn't a clue about using our computer.

"Aren't you typing your book on the computer?"

"If the guys turn it on and get it to the right screen, I'm usually okay, but there are too many confusing little pictures."

"Icons, Pam?"

"Yeah, I think Jon called them that. There are too many buttons and icons to accidentally hit, which messes everything up. Then I don't know how to fix what I've screwed up. The guys are never around when I need them, so I get horribly frustrated. It's easier writing longhand."

"Sure it is. How about e-mailing friends, Pam?"

"Rob set me up with an e-mail name, Lisa, so I could download all the lewd jokes my sister sends, but…"

"But what? When was the last time you checked your e-mail?"

"I refuse to answer on the grounds it may incriminate me."

"Pam…"

"All right. Rob showed me how to turn on the computer and plug into AOL about a month ago, so I checked it then. I forgot what he taught me, though, and I'm too embarrassed to tell Rob, because he thinks his mother is finally catching up to the rest of the cyber-world. Bill bought a laptop so I could write, but I can't figure it out. All I wanted was a cheap typewriter—something I could use to beat out a few letters and books. Is that too much to ask?"

"You could be e-mailing your friends on a daily basis, instead of never writing because you're too lazy to get out a pen and paper."

"All I want is a typewriter. Why is that such a terrible idea?"

"Do you remember what your papers looked like in college? If they were anything like mine, they were full of erasures and type-overs. Besides, you can't transfer information around with a typewriter, or save and delete it without reworking the whole manuscript. The computer makes life easier and more efficient."

"Oh, yeah?" I sniffed. "Rob tried to show me how to type on my laptop. Every time I touched the wrong button, my writing disappeared."

"It's usually not lost if you know how to retrieve it."

"Yeah, like I'm going to be able to figure that out." I rolled my eyes. I wondered how many others in this great world were as computer inept as myself?

"You have three children who could help you, Pam, or I'd be glad to show you how to work with the computer instead of against it. It's not your enemy, you know."

"It's easier to blame the computer than admit I'm a moron when it comes to technology."

"You know that isn't true. You're just resistant to machinery. You once told me you enjoyed working in the emergency room more than the intensive care units, because you hated taking the time required to under-stand the mechanical gadgets in the ICU."

"I hate machines. I should have been born a hundred years ago. Just out of curiosity, what's so bad about a handwritten letter anyway? It seems more personal to me. Everyone wants to jump on the computer to spit out letters."

"Handwriting is more personal, if you actually complete a letter."

"I'm terrible about writing letters."

"See? At least with e-mail, you can keep your notes short, sweet, and frequent. People might realize you haven't dropped off the face of the earth."

"Lisa, not only are you a wonderful cook, but you're a great listener. Thanks."

"You're welcome. Did you talk to Dr. Sitarik about herbal replacements to ease those miserable menopausal symptoms you're going to be facing soon and I'm not?"

"That's a cheap shot! But to answer your question, Dr. Sitarik wasn't too keen about them. He's seen no research investigating herbal stimulation of estrogen receptors in the breast, which is contraindicated with my type of cancer. I've made an appointment to speak with an herbalist, but I'm holding off on supplements for now."

"Planning any changes?"

"My diet is well-balanced, although I'm still working on chocolate. I eat loads of vegetables, and I always hoped that would even things out in the chocolate department. Based on my reading, however, I should cut out the little bit of alcohol I've always enjoyed." I cackled.

"What's so funny?"

"Ironically, since I was diagnosed with cancer, I've increased my alcohol consumption, but that's temporary."

"An occasional glass or two of wine won't hurt, Pam."

"Especially if it's red wine, which increases the heart protective cholesterol in the body. When I see patients with low HDL cholesterol, I tell them they can either exercise or drink red wine to increase it. Guess which most of them choose?"

"Ah. You're contributing to the alcoholic problem in this country."

"I guess it could be construed that way, but a little red wine goes a long way. Have you heard the joke about the patient who sees his doctor for a physical and is told that he must give up smoking, drinking, rich desserts, and women if he wants to live a long life? The patient says, 'If I give up all of that, what's the point in living?' "

"I've heard that one."

"I spoke with a nutritionist about dietary changes for cancer patients, Lisa. She encourages a well-balanced diet that is high in fiber and low in fat and emphasizes lots of anti-oxidants. She recommends veggies instead of anti-oxidant pills, because the interactions of anti-oxidants in foods are greater than the sum of the individual nutrients that are thrown into a bottle. I take a daily multi-vitamin and a couple of extra calcium tabs, since I'm a bit lactose intolerant. I'll add 1 mg of folic acid during chemotherapy, because it's supposed to decrease the incidence of mouth ulcers. Otherwise, I'm not planning any big changes."

"Uh huh. And how do you, with your frequent brain farts, remember to take your supplements?"

I beamed. "I have a handy-dandy seven day pill organizer. I just have to remember to separate the calcium tabs from the other pills to improve absorption."

"I wonder how long you'll stick to this regimen, Pam."

"Think you can't teach an old dog like me new tricks, huh? We'll see. I'm going to be compliant and stick with my routine."

"Compliant like the majority of patients who don't take all of their antibiotics or stop their blood pressure medications because they feel okay, or…" Lisa shot back.

"Okay, okay." I capitulated, holding up my hands in mock surrender to ward off the feigned attack. "I'll do my best, same as everybody else. But between you and me, I'm going to give this cancer one hell of a fight. I'm battling with everything I've got."

Chapter 13 - January 22nd

Dr. Sitarik's office looked dark and foreboding when I arrived for my first treatment—obviously a projection of my morbid mood. After my blood work was drawn, I sat in a deep, cushy loveseat reading bits of Gabriel Byrne's book, *Pictures in My Head*. Actually, I didn't absorb a single word, but I stared at the pages until I was called to an examination room.

A medical assistant, Laura, guided me to a scale. "Do I need to weigh myself every visit?"

"Yup. With this type of chemotherapy, it's not uncommon to gain ten to fifteen pounds. The doses of medications depend on your weight, and the doctors like to watch your progress. The nice thing is that we weigh you in kilograms, so unless you're pretty quick at conversions, it doesn't sound too bad."

"Terrific. I've spent eight months taking off nearly forty pounds and now I'm going to put on fifteen? I assume that's because steroids given to ward off nausea stimulate appetite."

"Ah, you read your handouts. That's right. That and the fact you tire easily and don't feel like exercising."

"Ha! I don't care how tired I get. I'll crawl on the treadmill if I have to, but I'm not gaining any weight back."

"Keep up that positive attitude, and you'll do fine. I'll take you to the examination room. Dr. Sitarik will be with you as soon as possible. He has an emergency admission, so it may be a while. But don't worry. The nurses will begin your chemotherapy no matter how late your appointment with the doctor runs."

"Great," I replied, meaning it. "The sooner I begin treatments, the sooner they will be over. I want to get on with the rest of my life."

Laura led me down a narrow corridor to an examination room. She gestured me inside, took my temperature and blood pressure, and recorded the information in my chart. Once the essentials were done, I wanted to acknowledge that I'd recognized her.

"I haven't seen you for a while, Laura."

"I didn't know if you would remember me, Mrs. Stockho."

"You didn't work in our office long, but you made a good impression. I hope you enjoy this job more."

"The pace is more relaxed, although the emotional stress is worse."

"I admire you. I don't think I could work in an oncology office every day."

"I miss working with you, Mrs. Stockho. I learned a lot from you." She smiled. "The doctor will be in as soon as he can. Would you like a magazine to read?"

"No, I always bring a book when I have a doctor's appointment. You never know what might come up."

Dr. Sitarik arrived twenty-five minutes later. "I'm sorry, Pam. I had an emergency admission."

"No problem. I know how emergencies can affect a full schedule."

After I undressed, Dr. Sitarik checked my lymph nodes, lungs, heart, and abdomen. "Your blood counts look fine, Pam. We can proceed with your first treatment today. As we discussed previously, I want you to lounge around the next three weeks. In ten days, I'll check a CBC to measure your white count and platelets. Remember you are most susceptible to catching infections between days ten to fourteen, so avoid anyone who is ill. We'll re-draw blood work on day twenty-one of the cycle and proceed with your second treatment on that day if blood counts are normal. Before each treatment, you will have blood drawn and see me for an examination. We'll review untoward effects you may experience. Most patients tolerate these particular drugs fairly well, so I don't anticipate too many problems."

Optimism temporarily thwarted my fear. A concrete plan was unfolding.

"Did anyone accompany you today, Pam?"

"No, I suspect I'll feel sorry for myself. I'm not great at small talk when I'm wallowing in self-pity. I plan to bury my despondency in an ice cream soda after my treatment."

"I wish I could join you for that ice cream. The first few hours shouldn't be bad, but you may experience nausea and fatigue for the rest of the weekend. Take it easy. Patients are often famished right after chemotherapy, secondary to the steroids."

I nodded.

"If you become terribly nauseated or vomit, I will call in an anti-emetic to your pharmacy. Keep the diet light this weekend, after the ice cream, of course."

"At least my kids and husband can fend for themselves. My husband is planning dinners for the week."

"Good man. Unless you have further questions, I'll turn you over to the treatment nurses. They'll answer concerns you have during therapy. I'll see you in ten days."

"Thanks." I shook his hand. "I want you to know I appreciate your bedside manner. This process is intimidating, and it helps to experience a little compassion."

I reluctantly trudged to the end of the hall, opened the door, and found myself in a large room. The colors echoed those of the waiting room. Light streamed into the room through a wall of glass. Eight recliners were arranged in a semi-circle—two provided the option of privacy curtains. Tables filled with Kleenex, straws, hard candies, IV supplies, and a sharps container for used needles stood adjacent to each chair. The walls were gray with splashes of purple and aqua. I inhaled the all too familiar hospital scents of alcohol and disinfectant.

"Hi!" a cheerful voice called out. "You look lost. You must be Pam Stockho, since everyone else scheduled today is an old customer. My name is Patty and I'm one of the oncology nurses. Pick any seat you would like— preferably one not presently occupied—and I'll be with you in a minute."

I looked around. There were four other patients, each with a companion. The patients were pale, bald, unsmiling, and hooked up to IV bottles. I sat next to a young couple taking turns reading from a Bible. The woman looked thirty-something. In spite of her bald head and pallid appearance, her face was stunning. She looked tiny and thin inside her red button-down shirt and blue jeans. A blanket covered her from the neck down but left exposed the port that had been placed in her left chest to ease venous access. An IV slowly dripped through it.

Although it had been offered, I refused a port since I had only six treatments to endure. The disadvantage was that a needle would be introduced into a vein in my right hand every three weeks. Since my surgeries involved my left arm and chest, I would need to avoid having blood pressures, blood draws, or IVs in that arm for now.

Patty busily prepared IVs, probably mine, so I studied the other couples. I wasn't nosy, but I loved observing people. Two of the other patients, a man and a woman, were older, probably in their late eighties or early nineties. I marveled at their decision to undergo chemotherapy at their ages. I wondered if I would have similar courage. On the other hand, I'd feel pretty good if I lived long enough to face that decision. Younger adults (probably twenty to twenty-five years older than myself) hovered near them.

A high school student sat to my left. A woman about my age kneaded his hand. He could have been my son. I was glad it was I, and not one of my children, facing this.

I focused on the mother's worried face—at least, I assumed she was his mother. The young man watched her. Suddenly, he bent down and rummaged through a canvas bag on the floor. He pulled out a brown paper sack, smacked his lips, and wolfed down a hotdog and chips. He washed everything down with a coke. Afterwards, he leaned his head against the back of the chair and closed his eyes.

"Sorry to have kept you waiting so long." Patty pulled up a stool. "Do you have a port or do I need to start an IV?"

"No port. But I don't think you'll have trouble finding a vein."

"Great. You wouldn't believe how hard it is to find a vein after a patient's had a few treatments. How many are you in for?"

"Six," I whispered as Patty patted my hand to raise a vein. I visualized myself as a prison inmate with her "how many are you in for" remark.

"I have ice chips for you to suck on for five to ten minutes before I push the 5-FU. The ice decreases the incidence of mouth sores. After I push the medication, I'll again ask you to suck on ice. You will receive three chemotherapeutic agents and two medications to prevent nausea. Did you review your handouts on side effects?"

I nodded, thinking back to the lists. More common side effects with 5-fluorouracil (or 5-FU) were sun sensitivity, mild changes in vision, diarrhea, nausea, low white counts, low platelet counts, hair loss, and mouth sores. Cytoxan (cyclophosphamide) could cause confusion, missed periods, fatigue, vomiting, anorexia, skin rashes, hair loss, chills, thirst, jaundice, and blood in urine or stools. In addition to many of the same side effects as the first two drugs, methotrexate might also cause abdominal pain, dizziness, headache, and edema. Actually, that list was more than I cared to remember. I put it out of my mind. If I developed side effects, I would deal with them as they arose.

"I've got your IV in, so let's get started." Patty hung a 50 ml bag of normal saline containing Decadron and Anzemet for nausea. As the IV ran in, I opened *Pictures in My Head* and read my favorite story—about the day Gabriel and his mother brought home his newborn brother; I needed to smile. I had read the book a couple of times, but today I just needed material that would numb my fears. I doubt I could have assimilated anything too profound.

After the IV finished, Patty hung another 50 ml bag of normal saline that would be used to flush the IV line, as drugs were slowly introduced directly into my vein. "Now we're ready to do your push meds." Patty showed me the syringes marked with my name and the amount of drug in each.

"I'm ready," I told her hesitantly, but as I watched Patty push the first chemotherapeutic agent, the first toxic chemical, through the IV catheter in my hand, I choked up, felt tightness in my chest, and cried. Dear God, please help me get through this. After Patty finished pushing the methotrexate and 5-FU, she started a slow infusion of the Cytoxan, which had been diluted in 250 ml of normal saline.

"The Cytoxan will take about an hour or so to drip in. Please let me know if you experience any sinus pressure. If you do, we'll slow it down a bit. I'm going to get you a blanket. Next time you come in, feel free to bring something to eat or drink." She squeezed my hand. "I can see how upset you are right now. It's understandable. I'll be right here if you need anything."

I nodded. My throat felt so constricted I couldn't answer her. My tears were embarrassing. Compared to being a patient, being a health care provider was easy. Most days at the office ended in a sense of fulfillment, especially when I had been able to help patients through some troublesome problems.

Before I broke my arm patting myself on the back, however, I had to admit I hadn't always been as sympathetic at home. Mentally exhausted each night, I wanted to believe everything at home would run smoothly. Ha! Over the past several weeks, however, I'd found fewer faults with our messy house and gave more time to hugs, dog walks, and letters—renewing acquaintances of friends long ignored except for Christmas cards.

As the drug dripped into my vein, I willed each cancer cell to explode. I pictured imperfect cells in my mind, watched the chemotherapeutic agents seep into the cytoplasm, imagined swelling and explosion of cell walls, and pictured white blood cells standing by ready to devour the refuse. I hoped the majority of exploding cells would be cancerous and not healthy ones. Interestingly, the more cells I pictured self-destructing, the lighter my heart felt. Burn, baby, burn, I repeated over and over. My mind visualized cancer cells burst into flame.

I had taken care of many dying patients, but I never thought about my death—me personally, *numero uno*. Now death boldly laughed at me, forcing me to face my mortality.

I watched the steady drip, drip of the IV. My brain felt very fuzzy, and I strolled along a beach, dragging my IV pole beside me, stopping at times to pick up shells and bits of seaweed. Patty strolled alongside me, whispering, "Pamalla". My eyes opened.

"You fell asleep," Patty said. "It's time to take out your IV and let you go home."

I made an appointment to see Dr. Sitarik and have blood work in ten days. I numbly left the office. Getting into my car, I drove down Broadway, past the Pearl Street Mall where Ben and Jerry's Ice Cream Parlor beckoned, but an ice cream soda no longer enticed me. I headed for home, parked the car in the garage, walked into the bathroom and examined my face, which was the color of a lemon. I cried so hard I threw up.

Chapter 14 - January 28th

I'd had a rough weekend, with bouts of nausea and depression. Rob set up a small television in my bedroom and I'd absorbed myself in movies, writing letters, sleeping, and playing with the dogs. With three dogs and me stretched out on our king-sized bed, there was little room for Bill. He gallantly offered to sleep downstairs, and I slept without earplugs for the first time in years. The dogs loved the attention, and they stayed by my side for two days—except at mealtime.

Before I started chemotherapy, I'd optimistically made a hair appointment with Kari at the Crazy Horse II Salon in downtown Louisville. It would still be a few weeks before I might begin losing hair and, although I could make that statement objectively, my gut wrenched every time I thought about the possibility of going bald. I didn't have one of those faces so gorgeous that hair was considered a complementary option. Nurse Patty, at Dr. Sitarik's office, had explained that with CMF chemotherapy, the odds of keeping most of my hair was in my favor, but I could experience quite a bit of thinning. It was Adriamycin that guaranteed baldness—a drug usually reserved for more aggressive or widespread tumors.

The thought of getting my hair cut made me feel normal. Actually, after the first couple of days following my treatment, I didn't look any different when I glanced in the mirror—the pasty, yellow facial tinge subsided. Putting on a bit of make-up, wearing nice clothes, and preparing to cut my hair provided the illusion I was as ordinary as everyone else. Ordinary was good.

I parked on Front Street and headed into the Crazy Horse II. Kari gave me a friendly wave. She was always cheerful, despite suffering chronic neck and shoulder pain. She wasn't going to be able to put off surgery indefinitely, but she hoped for a short reprieve from the pain with massage therapy.

Taking my jacket, she said, "So you're finally going to do it? You're going to let me wash that gray right out of your hair?"

"I am, Kari. I need a change. Actually, I'm experiencing more changes than I am interested in right now, but this one is positive. This one I am doing for me."

A puzzled look crossed her face, but she said nothing. That was one thing I loved about Kari. She would chatter away if a client was in the mood, but she also respected one's privacy.

"You've got on a beautiful sweatshirt, Pam. There shouldn't be any risk with the dye, but just to be safe, why don't you take it off, since you wore a denim shirt underneath?"

Oh oh. My breast and axillary pain had improved considerably during the month since my surgery, but getting my arm out of a sweatshirt still took a lot of effort. Pain continued to prevent me from reaching above my shoulder, and I wore three bras to walk on my treadmill and two at all other times to support my healing breast. I tried, unsuccessfully, to hurriedly remove my sweatshirt.

"Kari, if you don't mind, I could use your help getting my arm out of my sweatshirt. I had a bit of surgery about a month ago, and I'm still having trouble. Thanks."

I would have chuckled had I not been in pain. Calling what I was going through just "a bit of surgery" was like asking a patient if he had any chronic problems and being told, "Nah, I'm healthy. I had a touch of brain cancer once upon a time, but nothing serious."

Without comment, Kari helped me remove my arm from my sweatshirt and produced hair color samples from which I could choose the new me. I hadn't been blond since childhood, and I'd never pictured myself as a redhead, so Kari steered me toward my own natural color, albeit a shade or two lighter. The woman was an artist and a keen observer of human nature. She knew what would keep me comfortable.

While she mixed the color, I read a chapter in a book my friend Eilish had leant me: *Are You Irish or Normal?* Since I boasted no Irish heritage, I decided I must be at least borderline normal, a thought that comforted me momentarily. Other than reading in the beauty shop, I'd have precious little time to peruse humorous books today. After my hair appointment, I was meeting Eilish for lunch, and later, Gloria Bachelder was stopping by for a visit with her rambunctious two-year-old, Nicholas. He was always a delight.

I didn't often wish for grandchildren, at least no more than three or four times a day, but when I was around Nicholas, I pictured myself with a grandchild or two bouncing up and down on my leg playing horsey. My dad used to play horsey with us, and I remember laughing so hard I was close to throwing up—not a pleasant image for an adult, but as a child, being close to puking from laughing was way cool. However, I also knew where grandchildren came from, and as my three children were far from ready to become parents, I had to put those thoughts on hold for a few years.

Kari was ready with the goo. After raking it through, "to allow a little of the gray" to peek between chestnut brown-tinted locks, I sat with the concoction on my head for thirty minutes, entertaining myself by writing letters to friends.

I was working furiously on my third letter when Kari motioned me toward a sink to rinse and wash my hair. "You have such beautiful, thick hair," she said. I sobbed hysterically.

Poor Kari. She looked as if she'd been struck by a two-by-four. "What did I say?"

"I'm going to lose my hair, Kari. I have breast cancer, and I'm going to lose my hair soon."

"I thought it might be something like that," she said quietly. "When you had trouble with your arm, I wondered if that was the problem. I've known a few women with breast cancer."

Through my tears, I looked up at her expectantly.

"They're doing great."

I sighed.

"You're going to do great, too, Pam. I know you are."

"Thanks, Kari. You're a great morale booster."

"You're entirely welcome."

I left the Crazy Horse II less gray and happier of spirit thanks to Kari.

•••

I met Eilish through her lovely and energetic daughter, Katie, who worked college vacations in our clinic. I'd told Katie that I'd begun work on a novel about my breast cancer and planned on making the heroine— victim would probably have been a better term—an American of Irish descent. I had read quite a few books about Ireland, but I was not impudent enough to assume I had even the faintest hint of understanding the Irish people. I thought my first book could touch on Ireland, and I'd read loads more before embarking on my goal of setting a book in that island country. Of course, before I surrendered myself to composing such a fantasy, I fully expected to have visited Ireland. Bill had promised, now hadn't he?

I really enjoyed Eilish. She was quiet and refined, patiently answering endless questions about Irish customs and Irish history. She never made me feel stupid, despite some of the ignorant questions I posed. Eilish hailed from County Tipperary. She hadn't lived there in many years, although she visited frequently. Eilish was about my age, so information garnered on Ireland from her youthful perspective revolved around the 1950s and 1960s. Over several months, I began to understand what life had been like for Eilish as a child.

I walked over to the Old Louisville Inn, affectionately known as the O.L.I., which abutted the Crazy Horse II Salon. Hanging outside its door was an Irish tricolor flag. The pub offered a multitude of Irish culinary concoctions, many of them cooked/steeped/or battered in Guinness. Eilish hadn't arrived, so I picked a booth and allowed myself to become lost in the spirit of the place. I learned a bit about its history, thanks to the paper placemat cum history lesson set before me. The twenty-eight foot cherrywood and mahogany Brunswick back bar sported a copper trough, whose purpose, until I read my history lesson, had never been clear to me. The trough had accommodated miners' spitting tobacco!

Cigarette flames could have set off explosive mine gasses, so miners substituted chewing tobacco during working hours. While they sipped beers or threw back shots of bourbon after work, they occupied their mouths with their chew of choice. According to my O.L.I. history lesson, underground tunnels connected twenty-two bars in our town during Prohibition in the 1920s. I hadn't been able to verify the existence of the tunnels in any other Louisville document, but I liked the thought of all those miners pitching in together. Of course, drinking (and maybe tunnel digging) led to other pleasures, and the O.L.I. had boasted a brothel in the back (now a pool hall).

Three Colorado wildlife murals graced the walls of O.L.I. The primitive paintings were completed over a several day period in the 1940s by Cheyenne, a local artisan, who bartered the artwork for a running bar tab. The murals were uncovered during renovations in the 1970s.

Fixed to a far wall, an old tin sign proclaimed, "Guinness for Strength". I decided a pint would warm me up. In view of my resolve to decrease alcohol consumption, the decision to have a pint might have been construed as my lacking willpower, but I'd been led to believe that Guinness was more of a meal than a drink. It wasn't a beverage I consumed with regularity, but I enjoyed it occasionally.

By the time my pint arrived, so had Eilish, and we checked out the menu before I barraged her with questions. It had taken a few visits to the O.L.I., as well as the purchase of an Irish dictionary, before I learned how to pronounce the words emblazoned on the menu's cover that offered one hundred thousand welcomes to visitors: *Céad Míle Fáilte* (kayd **meel**-uh **fawl**-che). The Irish dictionary I'd bought boasted a confusing pronunciation guide. I was beginning to believe what I'd been told in jest—that the Irishmen who'd set down the spellings for what had been a spoken language were a bunch of mean-spirited drunks.

I ordered a plate of Guinness seasoned shrimp and chips, and Eilish, good woman that she was, ordered a salad. While we waited for our meals, I whipped out my ever-present list of questions about Ireland, and as usual, Eilish generously enlightened me. She whetted my appetite for more information about Irish counties' roles during the country's War of Independence (January 1919-July 1921) and the Irish Civil War (June 1922-May 1923). The Irish War of Independence united brothers, whose aim was to rid the country of England's heavy-handed rule. The Anglo-Irish Treaty of 1922 cleaved those same families as sure as it provided for a divided Ireland and a final blow to the pride of a people weary of tyrannical rule: a requirement that all swear allegiance to Britain. Brothers, once united, bent on destroying one other. Their fighting reminded me of our own Civil War, when families divided, interestingly, over the same group of people.

She shared a bit about activities in Tipperary of the Black and Tans, ruthless British ex-military troops who were sent to Ireland during the War of Independence to re-enforce local police. However, they failed to confine their inhumane tactics to criminals. Law-abiding citizens found their properties looted and riddled with bullets. Many innocents forfeited their lives— scenes echoed throughout the country.

Turning to less globally painful thoughts, Eilish asked, "How are you getting on with your treatments, Pamalla?"

"The first treatment could have been worse, Eilish. And I do have three weeks off, although I would gladly trade every day off for the next five years if I could wipe out what's happened since December."

"Are you getting some help at home?"

"I am. I've barely lifted a finger the last week or so, but I'll soon start cleaning closets and drawers. We've lived in Colorado for four years now, and I've longed to dispose of junk as we did before each military move."

"Have you joined a cancer support group, Pamalla?"

"It's not for me, Eilish. I'm not ready to share my feelings and trials with people I don't know. Besides, I spend every day at work listening to people's sad stories. I try to fill my leisure time with happiness. I've got friends, family, and myself, and I've made that elite group my support system. It works for me."

"That's all right then. As long as you have the support you need."

"I do. Thanks. How's Katie doing?"

"Ah, she's fine. She's planning a semester of study in Scotland."

"What fun. Maybe she'll return with a lovely Scotsman, like her dad, for a husband."

"I'll just be glad when she graduates from college."

"It will be a great loss to the clinic when she graduates and leaves us permanently."

"That's kind of you to say, Pamalla. She enjoys working in the clinic very much."

"I wouldn't have met you had it not been for Katie."

"That's true enough."

After lunch, I took the dogs for a walk. It would still be nearly two hours before Gloria and Nicholas arrived, so I popped in my favorite "feeling self-righteous and why-can't-we-care-more-about-each-other" movie, probably brought on by talk of Irish wars and a pint of Guinness: *Into the West*.

···

"Miss Pam!"

"Hi, Nicholas. How are you?"

He mumbled a few rapid words in his unique language, understood only in part by me and completely by his attentive mother, Gloria. She clutched a bouquet of flowers and a huge box.

"What's all this?" I asked, holding the door open for them.

"A few gifts to cheer you up and let you know we care about you."

I put the flowers in water as Nicholas made a beeline for the Brio train pieces I'd brought up from the basement. I hadn't kept many of the children's toys, but the wooden train that fascinated them all as small children still fascinated the next generation of rug rats. Noisily, he dumped train and railroad pieces onto the floor while he chattered contentedly. Every so often Gloria made what must have been an appropriate remark, because he'd listen attentively, smile, say something in Nicholas-ese, and resume his play. Before long, there was one two-year-old and two mommies playing with the wooden train.

"We miss you at the clinic, Pam," Gloria said quietly. "Everybody's asking about you."

"I miss you guys, too. I feel guilty having time off."

"You have nothing to feel guilty about. Don't worry about work, for goodness sake. We'll take you any way we can get you."

"It's great knowing I don't have to worry about being fired. I'm going to be away from work several weeks out of the next four months."

"No chance of getting fired. Everyone is just anxious for you to feel better. Your patients have been calling."

"I can guess which ones have been calling the most."

"You'd probably be right."

"You docs are afraid that if I don't return, you'll be saddled with the patients you've foisted on me."

"That's it exactly."

"There aren't many of those patients, are there? Most of our patients are grand."

"They are, and they've been asking when you're coming back. Most of them think you're on a fabulous vacation."

"Don't I wish!" Gloria handed me the box she'd brought, and Nicholas helped me unwrap it. Inside, a lilac sachet was nestled in an ecru silk nightgown and matching fleece robe. "They're beautiful, Gloria! Thank-you."

"You're welcome. When you're going through what you are, it's nice to surround yourself with beautiful things to wear. There's something else in the box."

And there was. Under the robe was a gift certificate to Essentials Spa in Boulder. "How can I Thank you?"

"Enjoy yourself as much as you can right now. And hurry back to us when you're ready."

Now how could I not get better with friends like that?

Chapter 15 - January 29th

I came from a small family. My mother had no siblings and my father, only one. I had four first cousins, but I couldn't remember the last time I saw them. My aunt and uncle died long ago. Interestingly, my uncle was Irish—last name of Dwyer—but that didn't count for me.

My sister, Linda, my only sibling, was a year younger than I, and growing up, she frequently paid for having a sister who received mostly A's in her studies. Mind you, I worked hard, and she often couldn't have cared less about her schoolwork, but sometimes I wondered how much of that was a direct result of the nuns' comparing her to me. In parochial school, she invariably had the same teachers a year after I did.

Persistently, she endured, "Why can't you be more like your sister?" from the nuns. That would have driven me batty. It's been said birth order can matter in one's personality development, and in situations like Linda's, I'd agree. On the other hand, being the older, I got stuck with the name nobody spells right—Pamalla. Firstborns often get saddled with weird names or weirder spellings. New parents probably never intend to drive their firstborns crazy, but it happens.

The constant harassment of the uncharitable Sisters caused Linda to hate school and me. My mother often said to us, "Just wait until you grow up. I hope you have fifty kids just like you." Linda didn't have kids, but she's had her revenge for following me in school. I got Linda's "I hate school" kid—Rob. I suffered every day he ditched class or refused to do his homework.

As Linda and I aged, our animosity vanished and love supplanted the rivalry—maudlin but true. We ran up phone bills that made the national debt look like a cheap date. Okay, since this is non-fiction, I'll admit that might be a slight exaggeration—slight.

We rarely lived near each other, thanks to Bill's far-reaching, bi-coastal naval treks. I flew home to North Carolina once a year, and two tours in Virginia made visiting home easier. One weekend during the first of those tours, Bill casually suggested (obviously without thinking about the implications of his generous offer), "Why don't you go down to your sister's for three or four days and I'll watch the kids?"

I spent the weekend lying in Linda's Jacuzzi tub and didn't think about Bill and the kids until my skin was as wrinkled as a prune's and in danger of sloughing off. And now that I think of it, Bill never made that offer again. That was actually the second time he'd magnanimously volunteered for kid duty. The first was when Heather was fourteen months old, I was pregnant with Jon, and I took the train down from New London, Connecticut, to the Big Apple to take a four day Lamaze instructor training course—four whole days. The man who had stopped smoking six months before was lighting up every ten minutes by the time I got back.

"How do you do it?" he cried.

How indeed, Moms? Most of us do it every day.

My call to Linda to tell her about my cancer was difficult. In fact, I spent some minutes talking to Linda's husband, David—who's an absolute gem of a guy—to see how he thought I should approach it. But Linda, listening to David's guarded side of the conversation, quickly realized something was seriously wrong and demanded the phone. Hey, just because she hated school and made lousy grades didn't mean she wasn't smart and intuitive—just like Rob.

"What's wrong with you?" she insisted. The shock of the news was readily evident by her momentary silence. Then she blurted out, "But there isn't any cancer in our family!"

Tell me about it, I thought. "Sometimes these things happen," I replied, more calmly than I felt. "I'm not happy about this either, but I can't wish it away. Believe me, I've tried. I thought you should know, but I wasn't sure when to tell you."

"I'm glad you called me. I want to see you. When's the best time to come?"

"You don't have to rush out, although I would love to see you. I don't look any different, although the new me is almost forty pounds lighter. You won't see any gross physical changes, like oozing pustules or boils—at least, I hope you won't. I'm willing my body to behave."

"I want, no, demand to see you," she said. "Name the date."

"I won't be working the next two weeks, so if there's any chance of your coming out the week of our birthdays, it would be ideal. Next week, my blood counts will fall, and I'm supposed to stay away from nasty, infected people; since you and I have a history of making each other sick..."

"Knock it off, girl," Linda laughed. "I'll arrive a week from tomorrow; that'll be the 6th. That way, we can celebrate our birthdays, and I can re-mind you that although we're both getting older, I'll never be as old as you are."

"Thanks. I appreciate your digging my grave a little deeper."

"You're welcome. Any chance one of the kids could pick me up at the airport?"

"You want to ride with one of them? You've mellowed."

"I'm getting old, kid, although, as I said, I'll never be as ancient as you. I'm dying to see you guys. Colorado looks so green in all the travel books."

"That's the other side of the Continental Divide. Except for our nearby mountains and the grass the natives put in, the terrain around here looks like western Kansas: dry, flat, and brown."

"Oh, doesn't that sound divine? Hmm. I guess instead of beauty, I'll have to settle for looking at you, the kids, dogs, and Bill."

"I think I've been insulted, Linda, but I'm not sure. If you want beautiful, we can drive up to the mountains."

"Fine. I'll call back later today with my flight number. Take care of yourself, kid. If anything happens to you, I won't have anyone but poor old David to torment."

"No, no, not that! Help me, please!" David hollered. The laughter escalated, so I said goodbye. I was already looking forward to her visit.

I made two more calls that night—one to my mom and one to my dad. Having been around longer than either Linda or me, they told me they knew I'd be fine, and somehow, hearing that, I believed I would.

...

"You're right, this part of Colorado is disgustingly flat and brown." Linda stared out the car window. "What's that nauseating smell?"

"We're passing odoriferous and scenic-challenged Commerce City. Sorry, but it's the most direct route home. It gets better." Linda rolled up her window to prevent further nasal bombardment from the stench of petroleum by-products and sulfur rising from the South Platte River.

"Louisville doesn't reek like this. Well, except in our house where you have to contend with the anal emissions of three males and three dogs. I will ask that you refrain from lighting matches in our house, since there is enough gas to spark an explosion."

"Thank God you have a daughter to remind you how cultured people behave."

"Are you kidding? Believe me, she can hold her own with the boys, and I will leave it at that. Between that and her perverted sense of humor, which she inherited from me, one never knows what to expect."

"And I wonder why I never had children, thank-you, God! I thought you'd send one of the kids to pick me up."

"I wanted you to arrive in one piece, so you're stuck with me." She seemed satisfied with that, gave me a little nod, and returned her attention to what passed for scenery.

The day was warm and the sky clear of the brown cloud of pollution that frequently settled over Denver. As I merged onto I-25 and headed toward Louisville, the majestic mountains known as the Front Range came into view.

"Linda, there's a ton of new construction between here and our little town of Louisville—lots of high tech. I'm hoping Jon will hire on with a local company after he graduates, but he's not promising. Heather has made it perfectly clear she's heading back to the beaches, and Rob wants to join the Army after high school. In a few years, I'll be experiencing empty-nest syndrome. Yes, yes! Make it so!"

"You're not in a hurry for the kids to leave home, are you, Pam?"

"Not really, but the illusion that my house may one day be free of kid droppings fills me with ecstasy."

"First kids, then grandkids."

"Oh, no, Linda, not for a while. And don't give Heather any ideas. The last time I brought up the subject of grandchildren, she didn't have a boyfriend. She looked at me, patted me on the arm and said, 'You want grandkids? Well, just let me know when. Give me ten months to produce, though, because I don't have any prospects for a father.' What a kid! I prayed for a year that she was kidding. No, I'm willing to wait.

"I adopt kids in the clinic. My favorite is an Italian charmer named Vinny. I can't keep my hands from running through his blond curls. He's only three-years-old, but he's smart as a whip. He was born on St. Patrick's Day, and every birthday he gets a St. Patrick's Day T-shirt from Bennigan's. I can picture the day when he decides it's time to stop with the shirts and begin with the pints of Guinness."

I glanced at the Flatirons as I got off the interstate in Louisville. Those mountains were about the last vestiges of undefiled terrain in our area. When we bought our home, the land around the interstate was inundated with prairie dogs, but growth forced their relocation. Now, there were few prairie dogs except those residing around housing developments, and the settlers in *these here parts* were not enamored of the cute furry critters, since they tunneled and made a *dang mess*. Personally, I loved them, but that was easy to say when one didn't have to fight for yard rights with them. At least they weren't skunks, although there were a few of *those critters* around as well.

I loved Louisville. It preserved many original buildings, thirteen of which were registered historical landmarks. The old section of town reminded me of one of those Hollywood Western sets, albeit with paved streets. Horses shared the roads with joggers, bicycles, Fords and BMWs. Farmers settled the area in the 1860s, and the town flourished after coal was first mined in 1877. By the 1890s, the area was populated by diverse groups of immigrants, including families of Italian, Austrian, Canadian, German, French, Scottish, English, Welsh, and Irish descent. Every time miners forged bonds to coerce humane treatment by their bosses, mine owners shipped in another ethnic group who would be less likely than veteran miners to strike.

Anticipating Linda's arrival, I'd borrowed books from the Louisville Public Library and stopped in at the Louisville Historical Museum to talk to its enthusiastic curator, Carol Gleeson. Many descendants of original mine workers still lived in our town. They donated time, antiques, and historical documents to restore and enrich the two museum buildings that began life as a store and three-room miner's house (circa 1904). Before Linda returned to North Carolina, I was determined to enlighten her on the history of our little town. I could hear her groan already.

The day after her arrival, I encouraged Linda to sleep late. In her world, late meant five a.m. I'd kept my mouth running the evening before for hours. The poor woman could scarcely get a word in edgewise with my motor mouth droning on and on. I even chased Bill out of the room.

After breakfast, Linda and I drove to Boulder. It was relatively warm for early February. I pointed out areas of interest, including the CU campus buildings and surrounding parks. We left our car in the parking garage on Spruce Street and hoofed it to Pearl Street Mall, one block away. Crossing at the light, I chilled. The winds had been increasing in strength all morning. There were times the winds along the Front Range approached one hundred miles per hour. There were many nights I lay in bed listening to the house creaking and windows rattling, and that wasn't always the aftermath of Bill's snoring. I hoped high winds wouldn't spoil our outing.

The ill feelings I suffered after chemotherapy had all but vanished, and I ecstatically embraced the mild winter day. Linda and I stepped onto the bricked walkway of the Pearl Street Mall. Someone with an artistic flair had placed a flower in the outstretched hand of a young girl forever captured in bronze by sculptor George Lundeen. Advertisements and circulars covered the poster pillars strategically placed down the center of the walkway, calling attention to upcoming local festivities and garage sales. Pearl Street Mall always reminded me of a European street, although it lacked Europe's omnipresent outdoor toilets.

It would be a couple of months before sleeping tulip bulbs would burst through flowerbeds that ran along the promenade, bringing color to the stark winter setting. In contrast to the bleak flowerbeds, smiles illuminated the faces of shoppers and pedestrians leisurely strolling the jammed walkway. I guided Linda through favorite shops as we made our way to Rocky Mountain Joe's Café for lunch. Kiosk owners had braved the elements to sell their wares, which ranged from hotdogs and Caribbean food to whimsical hats and handmade jewelry.

We opted for indoor seating overlooking the mall. I loved eating outdoors, but my usual cold intolerance had increased since chemotherapy. It was probably secondary to my decreasing cell count and relative anemia. We ordered Mediterranean salads. Linda stared at me to the point of making me uncomfortable. I stared back.

"You seem to be handling this pretty well, Pam. I would be falling apart."

"I have good days and bad days. I try to keep bad days to a minimum, although I never know when a feel-sorry-for-myself hour may hit. My lowest point so far was during my first treatment. I felt violated by chemotherapy. Odd that healthy me should be assaulted by toxic drugs, when I've never touched a joint, sniffed anything stronger than gardenias, and never ventured into the spiraling abyss caused by street drugs. I sat in the treatment room, telling myself over and over that chemotherapy was my best shot at eradicating this lousy cancer. It took a lot of convincing on my part—and more than a few tears as well.

"I tell myself I can fight with weapons available in my personal arsenal: resting, eating well, and maintaining a positive attitude, but in truth, I feel impotent in the battle. I am along for the ride and others control my destination. It's frightening."

"How are Bill and the kids holding up?"

"They're walking around with frayed nerves and tight lips. They want to help but don't know how. They feel more powerless than I do. I should be reaching out to them, but I can't. Not yet. I barely keep my emotions reined in as it is. I read an article years ago that claimed the odds of getting cancer were one in five. Those odds have probably changed, but at the time I prayed that if someone in our family had to suffer cancer, I hoped I would be afflicted rather than Bill or the children. Isn't that silly? I know that one in five odds doesn't mean that out of a family of five, one will definitely get cancer, but that didn't prevent me from praying. I remembered that plea the other day. I hope God protects my family."

Unexpectedly, Linda giggled.

"What are you snickering about? I could use a good laugh."

"Remember when we lived in Germany, Pam?"

"I remember wheeling our doll carriages through the cemetery across from our apartment."

"I was more interested in pushing little boys in the dirt than pushing baby carriages. You might recall I was the family tomboy."

"I remember, Linda."

"Do you remember older brothers of the boys I pushed in the dirt coming around to beat you up when it came time for retribution, Pam?"

"How could I forget? A bloody nose out of the blue, a punch to the abdomen and the scurrying of feet in the opposite direction."

"I was so scared the time I found you passed out in the basement. That must have been one terrible blow to the stomach."

"I was only six, for goodness sake. I could take it better now. You were something for a five-year-old, Linda. Nobody could scramble up a tree faster than you."

"True. I thought I was brave then, but you're the brave one now. I admire you."

"Don't admire me too much, kid. I can't walk away from this. I'm stuck, so I'm doing the best I can, despite the emotional roller coaster that keeps me spinning out of control. I always wanted to win the lotto—be a big winner in a contest where the odds were against me—but this isn't the lotto I wanted to win." I sighed. "Enough sadness. I'm in the mood to spend a little cash. Let's visit stores at this end of the mall."

While we walked, I caught up on gossip from home. "How's Mom doing, Linda?" My mother spent a lot of time at Linda's house. Mom created breathtaking arrangements from silk flowers and seed pods, and Linda and I were the happy recipients of Mom's creativity. Linda and Mom spent a couple of days each season decorating my sister's house. Eat your heart out, *House and Garden*! Linda and decorating weren't the only reason Mom spent a lot of time at my sister's place. The resident cocker spaniel, Maggie, had charmed her way into Mom's heart. Maggie was the granddog Mom always wanted, because she lived nearby.

"Mom and I spent the weekend cooking, Pam. We had a ball."

"Gross! How you two can enjoy preparing meals is beyond me. I still can't believe you took Chinese cooking classes. The only cooking classes I'd be willing to enroll in would be entitled, 'How to get out of cooking for your family'."

"You missed out on some delicious egg rolls, kiddo."

"You didn't bring me any, by some chance, did you, Linda?"

"Sorry, no, but I'd be glad to send the recipe."

"You've got to be kidding! Save the postage. Is Pop still creating savory dishes in Myrtle Beach?" Dad lived in South Carolina and Mom lived in North Carolina. They had separate lives and were the happier for it.

"Dad loves to cook as much as I do. I have no idea where you inherited your hate to cook gene, but the rest of us love it."

"I don't think I'll change. I know as little about creating meals as possible. Thank God Heather loves to cook. If I'd been a bit more enamored of the kitchen, I might not have made such a fool of myself when I learned to suture."

"What do you mean, Pam?"

"Years ago, one of the docs I worked for in Virginia Beach suggested I get some pigs' feet to suture, because closing cuts on pig skin is about the same as suturing lacerations on human skin. How was I to know that I could have bought fresh pigs' feet? I bought macerated, pickled pigs' feet and spent several frustrating hours trying to suture pieces of skin that literally fell apart in my hands."

"You didn't!"

"I did."

"And YOU got straight A's in graduate school, Pam?"

"I have my limits."

"Obviously." She laughed hysterically, and I decided to put off more questions about life in Fayetteville and Myrtle Beach until later.

My favorite shops along the Pearl Street Mall featured works of local artisans. I admired metalworkers, sculptors, painters, quilters, jewelers, knitters, woodworkers, and basically anyone with talented hands. I had no gifts in that area. Linda and I wandered through the Boulder Arts Co-op. I settled on a couple of Alan Klug photographs taken in Ireland: an old bicycle—its woven basket teeming with pink flowers—leaning against a church window; and a thatch-roofed white cottage fronted by a bright blue door in County Galway.

How was it that photographers like Alan Klug and Jill Freedman saw the same things I did, but envisioned so much more, brilliantly capturing the pure essence of subjects on photographic paper? I paid for my prizes and walked out, Linda on my heels. She'd picked up a photograph of the Flatirons. I was winning her over to Boulder County, Colorado; believe me, based on the number of people pouring into the area, that wasn't difficult.

On the way to the car, we stopped to admire the Boulder Courthouse, which was erected in the 1930s to replace the fire-gutted structure that previously served the city. The amber colored façade was elegant, sharply contrasting with the shabbily clothed indigents who spent their days lolling on the front lawn. A few strummed old guitars, beat drums, or shared a few words.

The clothing and hairstyles of Boulder's poor reminded me of hippies from the 1960s. Barring freezing temperatures, they were omnipresent on Pearl Street Mall. When we moved to Boulder County, I felt uncomfortable being confronted with stark poverty when my goal was to spend a few bucks in stylish boutiques and fashionable cafés. But my discomfort was appropriate, and since then I always shared a few dollars with those in need.

Linda and I stopped at the Renegade Rose Flower Shop. I chose a glorious spring bouquet to nurture my spirit before venturing outside once more to combat the increasing wind. Our coats whipped around our legs as we edged toward my favorite card shop, The Printed Page. Besides cards, there were books, paintings, art supplies for children, and other delightful diversions intent on putting a significant dent in my wallet. The sales clerks carried on a light-hearted banter.

"You're making fun of me," one jested.

"Well," countered the other, "you always say I'm not a nice person, and you do make it easy to find fault with you."

"You can be so mean at times," the first clerk retorted, with just a hint of a smile, "but at least you're always available to work when I need you."

"You know I'm here for you," spoke the second. "Besides being mean to you, I live only to serve you." She rang up my purchases. The smile never left her face—or mine.

We stopped at the Boulder Bookstore before heading home. If I ever tired of nursing, I could happily run a small bookshop and cater to my inner child. I could imagine myself sitting among stacks of novels and non-fiction tomes, helping a high school student find historical material for an assigned paper, or assisting a grandparent choose the right tale for her grandchild.

I left Linda in the romance section of the bookstore while I searched through Irish history and travel books. I was deeply involved in a lovely little book called *Of Irish Ways* by Mary Murray Delaney, when a firm rap on my shoulder startled me.

"I'm ready when you are," Linda announced innocently. She glanced at the floor around my feet. "Are you buying ALL those books?"

"Yes, I'm buying them all."

"I found two romance novels I haven't read yet."

"Grand." I hoisted my stack. We waited in line for several minutes while clerks assisted other shoppers. I never minded waiting in bookstores. There was always something in my hands to read.

We turned the corner beyond the Boulder Bookstore as the clouds opened and delivered raindrops the size of ping-pong balls.

"Where did that storm come from?" Linda demanded. "There wasn't a black cloud in the sky when we left home."

"Welcome to Colorado, Linda, my dear. The weather is as fickle as a married lover. Have a nice day."

•••

"Now where are we off to?" Linda asked.

"I'm dying to try on wigs, just in case..." I couldn't finish the sentence. I swallowed with difficulty.

Everyone's Hair in Boulder was a small beauty salon that advertised wigs for special people losing hair from chemotherapy. I wasn't sure the quality of the wigs would be any better, but I hoped there might be compassion behind that message. Tony guided me to a seat in a discrete, partitioned area. He encouraged me to try on as many styles and colors as I wanted. With Linda barely able to keep a straight face, I tried on wigs with

118

short curls and long tresses. I tried bouffant styles ("I look like Marge Simpson.") and pixie cuts.

I'd been right when I told Kari I could no longer pass for the blond I'd been in my youth. Bright red hair was definitely not in my future, and jet-black tresses bleached out my facial coloring so much I resembled a corpse. In the end, I opted for a wig with coloring very much like my own pre-gray tresses—not unlike the color Kari steered me toward when she dyed my hair. I noted the style and color and assured Tony I would return if my hair fell out dramatically. Believe me, verbalizing that statement took effort. I never fancied myself a female Telly Savalas, bald as a baby's bottom, although I could visualize myself strutting around with a Tootsie Roll Pop asking, "Who loves ya, baby?"

"Now you take care of yourself," Tony encouraged. "I've seen a lot of patients with cancer. The ones who do best drink protein shakes and power lounge."

"Power lounge?"

"Power lounge. Relax, put your feet up, and meditate each day. Let the world come to you for a change. I hope all goes well for you."

"Thanks for the tip, Tony—and the encouragement. Have a nice afternoon."

...

Linda and I spent several glorious days power lounging. We sprawled on chaises we dug out of the garage. The weather was intermittently warm. On colder days, Linda indulged me in watching Irish movies like *Michael Collins, My Left Foot, The Commitments, High Spirits,* and *The Secret of Roan Inish.* We romped with the dogs in area parks. We read books, shopped, and visited friends.

The days raced by. Linda would be leaving in a handful of days, and I would receive my second chemotherapy treatment before she left. I felt guilty I'd failed to plan exciting activities for her. We'd spent a day in the popular section of Denver known as LoDo, took in a show at the Comedy Works, shopped, and walked along the outdoor Sixteenth Street Mall. But I could have bought tickets to the Colorado Ballet, Opera Colorado, or the Boulder Dinner Theater, to name a few. To be honest, I had enjoyed doing nothing but relaxing, spending the week with one of my best friends. I gave voice to my guilt.

"Do I look upset?" Linda asked. "Do you have any idea how long it's been since I had the opportunity to sit around and do nothing and not feel guilty about it?"

"How about a trip to Breckenridge today?" I probed while she ate her breakfast and perused newspaper clippings I'd collected about Colorado.

"Which highway goes into the mountains from here?"

"I-70."

"This I-70?" She shoved the paper under my nose.

I scanned the front page. An SUV had been crushed under more than a ton of rocks. Rains had loosened stones from up to a half-mile from the highway. More than seventy-five boulders had spewed down the mountainside, smashing the vehicle and killing the occupants. It had been the worst rockslide in history to date.

"That would be the same I-70."

"Pass."

"But that type of catastrophe is rare! Highway workers spend hours scouring mountaintops for loose rocks."

"They obviously missed a few."

"There'd been a lot of rain. We'll be fine, honestly. Rockslides don't happen very often."

"Pass. I'll look at pictures of the mountains instead."

"Chicken. If you don't want to go to the mountains, you'll be forced to listen to me entertain you about the history of Louisville."

She groaned. "Those are my only two options?"

"Yup."

"I suppose you've done a lot of research to bore me."

"Tons."

She groaned again. "No mountains."

"Boy, are you going to be impressed by the amount of homework I've done."

"I can hardly wait." She didn't sound particularly excited.

The day was bright and warm, so we walked the two miles into the old part of town. "The weather can be crazy around here, Linda. It might snow this afternoon. We've had really nice days while you've been here. You must have brought good weather from North Carolina."

"I'm happy I could brighten up your dreary winter." We sauntered in silence toward old Louisville. The silent part was quite an accomplishment

120

for me. It wasn't totally quiet, however. Several Louisville canines seren-aded us.

"Most of these old houses are tiny," Linda remarked as we edged toward the center of town.

"Many were built for miners. The town was divided along ethnic lines for quite a while. Italians, who began arriving in the 1890s, were initially refused city water, and then they were forced to pay twice as much as everyone else. The city only allowed them to use water for two hours a day.

"Italian Catholics endured cross burnings in their front yards by the Ku Klux Klan in the 1920s. You'd think that as much as the men depended on each other in the mines, they would have learned to live peacefully together. They suffered through long strikes, lean times, and mine explosions, but the mine owners' practice of breaking strikes by hiring ethnic groups to cross picket lines kept men separated except during frequent street brawls. One fight, between an Irishman and a Canadian in 1882, lasted sixty-three rounds. I'll bet the Irishman would have won if the Canadian hadn't had ten years and twenty pounds on him."

"Where'd you come up with that stuff?"

"I found a couple of books in our local library: *Louisville Histories* that were collected by local school kids, and *The Louisville Story* by our eminent historian, Carolyn Conarroe. Just for you, I also pored over documents in the Louisville Historical Museum. Did you know mining was a seasonal occupation, Linda?"

"Nope, never knew that, Pam. But I suppose you plan to tell me all about it."

The woman knew me too well. She probably wasn't interested, but that didn't stop me from jabbering. She was usually a good sport, though, only sighing when she couldn't take any more of my shameless chatter. I was shy around people I didn't know well, so friends and family got more of me than they wanted. I could hear my nurse pal, Barb, laughing: "You—shy? Give me a break."

I cleared my throat. "The coal mined in Louisville was almost twenty per cent water. As it dried, it crumbled, so it couldn't be transported much farther than Denver. Spontaneous combustion precluded storing the coal for long, so mine operations were severely curtailed during the harsh part of the winter and the hot summer months."

"Aren't you a trove of useless information?"

"I am—and proud of it. There's more."

"I'm not surprised."

"I'll go easy on you."

"Thanks, mucho."

"Don't mention it."

"I won't." Linda stared at me, probably in shock that I planned to refrain from overwhelming her with a two-hour monologue. I reminded myself of priests I'd known whose protracted sermons put parishioners to sleep. I checked her eyes to make sure the lids weren't drooping.

"What?"

"Nothing, nothing. Making sure I'm not boring you to death."

"I'll be the first to let you know, Pam."

I sneered at her. She occasionally flipped through my copy of *The Louisville Story*, so she wasn't completely bored by our historical jaunt.

"Mrs. Conarroe signed this," Linda announced unnecessarily, since the author had graciously done just that when she met me for lunch.

"I'm moving up in the world, rubbing shoulders with authors. Next thing you know, I'll get Gabriel Byrne to sign his book for me."

Linda snorted. "Like that's going to happen. Pretty soon you'll tell me you're planning a trip to Ireland."

"As a matter of fact, Bill promised to take me after my treatments are over. I'm really excited."

She stopped perusing *The Louisville Story*. "That's great! I know you've been dying to go. Have you gotten your passport yet?"

"I haven't. I thought I'd wait until after my treatments are done."

"Oh. You mean when you're as bald as a cue ball?"

My mood soured. "Thanks a whole hell of a lot. Maybe I won't wait."

She stuck her nose back in the book. "There is definitely some interesting reading in this book."

We were standing outside the O.L.I. "This is the last of the original saloons that used to grace Front Street. Around 1900, there were thirteen bars in Louisville. The entire population of the town numbered just over one thousand. Sounds like the bar-population ratio one sees in small Irish towns, doesn't it?"

She failed to appreciate my attempt at humor, so I moved on. "During Prohibition, a number of illegal stills operated here, including one by an elderly woman. Her poultry did her in." There was a pregnant pause as I waited to suck Linda into my story.

"What happened?" she demanded. The woman loved my stories, even if she hated to admit it.

"Supposedly, the old woman mixed hooch ingredients in a barrel and then fed the corn remnants to her chickens. Their staggering around alerted police to her illegal shenanigans and her place was raided."

"You made that up."

"Did not!"

"Did too!"

"Nope."

We popped into the O.L.I. for a couple of sandwiches before continuing our tour of the town. A train whistle caught Linda's attention. "What's that?"

"The train tracks run just behind this pub. Without those tracks, there would have been no Louisville. It's a pain in the rear when traffic is backed up several times a day, but, hey, otherwise we might not be living here today. And I do so love this sleepy little town, parked between Denver and Boulder—the best of two very different worlds."

We walked off our lunch trudging to the Family Medical Center. I introduced Linda to the nurses, doctors, and staff. The sagging diaper that had graced the nurse's station was gone. Unfortunately, the saturated diaper had dropped during the night, and all bets were off. I spent a few minutes reviewing charts on my desk and made phone calls to patients who had left messages. Linda and I commiserated on the sorry state of my workplace. Her office building was just two years old, everything still in pristine condition.

"I miss this place," I said. "I haven't missed the tiny exam rooms and offices, but I miss the staff and patients. It's been wonderful, recharging at home for three weeks, but I'm ready to return to work. Too much time at home drives me crazy."

"And *I'm* ready to go home, Pam. Too much time with relatives, no matter how wonderful, can drive everyone crazy."

"How about Breckenridge tomorrow?" I asked. "After that, I'm having chemo again and you're going home."

"Will you guarantee there will be no rockslides on the way up the mountain?"

"I guarantee it."

"Fine. But I swear that if we die in some landslide, I'm going to murder you."

Chapter 16 - February 15th

Three weeks had passed since I graced the medical clinic I called home for forty-plus hours a week. I weathered my second chemotherapy treatment the Friday before with about as much charm and elegance as I'd displayed the first time. I had clutched *Pictures in My Head* like a security blanket, occasionally reading favorite Irish stories, during which I survived another round of intravenous meds before returning home—scared, nauseated, and jaundiced. I frightened Linda with my sallow complexion, so I smiled wanly and willed myself not to puke. She tucked me into bed and again berated me for not allowing her to accompany me to Dr. Sitarik's office. Truthfully, I'd been afraid I'd cry like I had the first time. I didn't. I acted like a big girl and read my book, with a warm blanket tucked around me to ward off chills. Besides, Linda had complained of a sore throat for twenty-four hours, and the last thing immune-suppressed patients needed was germs spewed all over them. So she stayed home and awaited my return, nursing me until it was time for Bill to take her to the airport on Saturday.

Three days after my treatment, I was a human being again—relatively speaking—and ready for work. I waved at staff members, who seemed happy to see me, as I trudged toward the infinitesimal office I shared with Dr. Richard. It seemed smaller than I remembered. I pulled my chair out and plowed into the poor doctor, who was sifting through stacks of charts on his desk.

"A weekend off and these charts multiply," he boomed. "They must be Catholic." Turning, he knocked into my chair and upended the wastepaper basket. "Pam, welcome back. We missed you."

"I'll bet you're thrilled to see me, doc. At least when I was gone, you had this cubbyhole to yourself."

"True, but no one to talk to while I labored over patient charts, and at least you're a captive audience when it comes to my jokes. How are you feeling?"

"Fine. Really. So far, I've only been sick for a couple of days after treatments."

"And you've had two so far?"

"Yes."

"You're a third of the way through chemo."

"Thanks for the positive thinking, doc."

"You're welcome. You've been off three weeks, and now I understand you want next week off too?" he chuckled.

"Yeah. I'm going to need one week of every chemo cycle off, 'cause you guys can make me sick."

"We do that when you're not receiving chemotherapy, so what's the big difference?"

We turned our attention to the messes on our desks. It was ten to 8:00 in the morning. None of my charts required immediate attention, and I never called patients before 9:30 unless it was an emergency. Pushing out my chair carefully to avoid hitting Dr. Richard again, I ambled to the front desk to chat with the staff. I spent a couple of minutes savoring the de-delighted smiles on young patients' faces as they pressed their hands and noses against our tropical fish tank. The fifty-gallon tank was recessed into a wall, protected on three sides from prying young hands.

"Sophia, whose turn is it to clean the fish tank? It looks like my car after the dogs snort all over the windows."

Sophia burst out laughing. "Welcome back. We missed you. And your patients really missed you. What should we tell them? Do you want to be sick, on vacation, what? Everyone thinks you've been on a glorious Caribbean cruise."

"I wish. I'll write up something for you to hand out. It shouldn't be your responsibility to make up excuses for me. I really don't mind if people know about my cancer, although I don't plan on announcing it to the world—at this point anyway. I'm sorry. I should have thought about that weeks ago."

"I'm sure patients were not foremost on your mind the past three weeks. Oh, and by the way, since everyone thinks you've had a lovely vacation, you can clean the handprints on the fish tank. Paper towels and glass cleaner are in the kitchen—not that any of you providers know how to clean anything around here."

"A little feisty this morning, aren't you? Busy?"

"It's Monday. What else is new? It's eight o'clock, and we only have three appointment openings left for the entire day. Dr. Bachelder is worried about you. She had us close your schedule this afternoon and plans to send you home at lunchtime. Per her instruction, we've booked you three patients an hour this morning until you see how tired you get."

"That's sweet of Gloria, but we need more openings for patients. If I don't see four patients an hour, the docs will have too many work-ins. Open up my schedule this morning. If I can't manage, I'll take extended leave and get someone to cover for me."

"That's what the doctors are worried about, Pam. They'd rather you see fewer patients an hour than have someone cover for you. They're willing to see extra patients to accommodate you for a few months. They figure you're worth it. The staff, on the other hand..." A huge grin lit up her face.

"It's great to be loved and appreciated, Sophia."

"Ha!" she replied.

I turned to Sophia's co-workers. "How are you today, Tricia and Laurie?" Among the three of them, charts were pulled, and patients were checked in and out.

Tricia, in particular, was a joy. She worked her fanny off. She transferred to our clinic after her previous employer literally worked himself to death. Tricia fit in perfectly, contributing her share of jokes and good-natured teasing to keep those staff members who enjoyed a bit of fun in good humor.

Our clinic had suffered a rash of turnovers at the front desk during the past few months, so we were fortunate she joined our team. Not everyone in our little town was pleasant to deal with, as unbelievable as that might seem, and the front desk personnel took the brunt of anger from patients ticked off about updating insurance information or waiting for appointments when providers got behind. Some folks were just unpleasant, and it took only one miserable human being to ruin your day.

Interestingly, the results of an informal poll I took years ago proved that the amount of anger generated by any patient was inversely proportional to the severity of his or her illness. And that held up through the years. Really sick patients seemed thankful to be seen and didn't waste precious energies screaming at medical staff.

Although Laurie, who was assigned to pull charts, didn't suffer the verbal tirades from patients that Sophia and Tricia did, the rest of us complicated her job. Charts were rarely filed appropriately, and none of us (myself included) consistently filled out the cards that indicated to what part of the office the chart had evaporated. Laurie invariably spent the better part of each day cruising the clinic, searching everywhere for charts. Somehow, she always found them.

I glanced at my watch. It was ten past eight, which meant my first patient was late, and the next couple of patients would have to wait for me to catch up. I walked back to my office. I had been very thankful when Dr. Richard offered me a home. Prior to that, I'd been a nomad, moving from office to office depending on which doctor had a day off. Four doctors and I shared four offices, and Dr. Hibbard vacated his office when his wife, Dr. Chris Hibbard, counseled patients two afternoons a week. Canned sardines had more room than the five of us regular providers crammed into four offices and eight exam rooms. We needed more space.

Providers worked four, ten-hour days to solve the space crunch. When someone was on vacation, or getting cancer treatments, the office worked short. Like other hardworking professionals, our physicians considered their time off sacrosanct. Occasionally, float pool nurse practitioners, physician's assistants, or doctors were employed to stem the overflow of patients. The drawback was that they didn't know our patients like we did, and our patients appreciated consistent care.

The clinic was so popular we needed five patient care providers every day, but we couldn't accommodate more than four. Two exam rooms apiece weren't enough when we had a couple of patients plugged into IVs and a couple of others receiving breathing treatments. The end result was a lot of overbooking, leading to exhaustion and frustration for all of us.

Like many clinics around the country, our family practice was purchased by a local hospital, Boulder Community. Clinics entered into long-term relationships with larger facilities to stave off bankruptcy. I knew what patients thought. When they saw the charges for a fifteen-minute appointment, they figured we were raking in the dough. What they didn't understand was that managed health care groups reimbursed only a fraction of the charge, forcing already overworked caregivers to see more and more patients, desperately hoping to stem costs spiraling out of control.

Dr. Richard plowed into the back of my chair as he swiveled in his seat to pick up a chart he dropped on the floor. "Oops, sorry, Pam. I didn't realize I was so far from my desk."

"You weren't, doc. You can't be very far from your desk in this room. Despite the cramped accommodations, I have to tell you I appreciate your sharing your office with me."

"Our office, Pam. And it's fine. Boulder Community promises a new facility, with more exam rooms. One of these days it's going to happen."

"We'll probably be cold and stiff before we see that day, doc. And how many years will it take to pay off a new building with reimbursement what it is?"

"No negative waves, please. Hey, want to see the newest batch of pictures taken of me at training camp?" Dr. Richard, a huge Rockies fan, had attended the past two Rockies' Fantasy Camps. His nickname was "Doc", and he even had occasion to practice his suturing skills. His 8X10 baseball camp pictures graced the wall of exam Room 2. Occasionally, he got a little behind when patients commented on the photographs. He regaled them with tales of his baseball exploits and physical prowess.

At twenty minutes past eight, I was summoned, via overhead pager, to see my first patient. "Pam, Room 5." I eased myself out of my chair to prevent hitting Dr. Richard and walked down the narrow corridor to the nurse's station.

Dr. Hibbard's rear end greeted me in the nurse's station. True to form, he was bent over a wastebasket, muttering, "How hard is it to separate single-layered cardboard from trash? And look at this—two soda cans. They can be recycled!" He stood, his hands full of recyclables. "Good morning, Pam."

"Morning, doc."

A true Boulderite, the good doctor made daily trashcan rounds in the clinic, salvaging recyclable cans, paper, and single-layered cardboard. The liberated objects found their way into carefully labeled bins in the backyard. Most of us did our part to protect the environment, but none of us was as dedicated as Dr. Hibbard. Some, including me, felt the man was obsessed. He took that as a compliment.

My thoughts turned to my morning schedule. Krystal was stuck working with me. Although a medical assistant, she knew as much about nursing as many of the R.N.s I'd worked with over the years. She made my job a whole lot easier, efficiently getting patients into rooms and rounding up appropriate equipment.

"Morning, Krystal." Since Barb usually helped me on Mondays, I asked, "How come you're not working with me today, Barb?"

"I begged for a reprieve, and God granted me one. I forgot you were coming back today and hadn't psyched myself up enough to deal with you."

"Funny, very funny, Barb!"

"I thought so. Seriously, Gail's off today, so I'm stuck with phone duty. And given a choice between working with you or getting screamed at by patients on the phone when I can't get them immediate appointments, which do you think I'd take?"

The phone nurse remained glued to a chair in the nurse's station for ten hours a day; the half-hour she got for lunch was rarely long enough to resurrect her sanity. She returned patient calls and triaged demands for same-day appointments once providers' schedules filled. She decided who needed to be worked-in on an emergency basis and who could wait to be seen for a day or two. She received an occasionally spirited, "Fuck you!" from irritated patients. She called in refills for medications and phoned patients with results of lab work and radiology reports on which providers had commented. Other nursing staff assisted the harried phone nurse whenever possible. The position rotated as often as possible, because the *phone queen for a day* took loads of verbal abuse. I tried to keep on her good side by calling my own patients. So for Barb to intimate she'd rather be the phone nurse than work with me...

"It's great to be back, Barb. I love the respect I get around here."

"Respect? You? I don't think so! Oh, by the way. Your patients all know you're back. You've got a stack of charts with phone messages sitting on the med refrigerator. I'll bet you can guess who half of them are from."

And she was right. I loved our nurses. We ragged each other regularly to relieve the tension. It worked for us. None of us took such comments personally, because our remarks were *never* mean-spirited. New staff members were always protected from our teasing until we knew whether she or he felt comfortable with our particular brand of humor. If someone didn't join in the fun, we respected that. However, I believe our humor kept many of us sane in our increasingly insane environment.

Actually, Barb and I had given each other hell for years. We traded many mother horror stories about her two teen-aged boys and my three kids. I told her once I longed for the kind of family where everyone sat around the table and got through an entire meal without someone telling a lewd joke that elicited a quick descent into belly laughs and inane behavior. Of course, since I usually started the jokes, I couldn't expect much, but just once, it would have been nice to have an intelligent conversation at the dinner table.

Barb had choked out, "Right! In *your* house? Miracles don't occur in your house any more often than they do in mine. Did I tell you about the time Ryan told a joke at dinner and laughed so hard he snorted milk out his nose?"

That was Barb and I. We'd never make it into the record books for mealtime decorum, but our kids loved us. Go figure.

"Pam, you gave Bert Everett samples of Accolate, right?"

"I did, Barb. How's he doing?"

"Great. He feels like a new man. His asthma is under control for the first time in years. He'd like a prescription."

"No problem."

"Actually, there is. Accolate isn't on his HMO's formulary. They require written justification."

"He's already on a short-acting bronchodilator, an inhaled steroid, a long-acting beta-adrenergic agonist, and a preventive inhaler. With the samples of Accolate I gave him, his asthma is under good control, and they want to know why we'd like to keep him on it? HMOs! Sometimes medical insurance companies drive me nuts. Do they think I prescribe expensive medications because I can't be bothered to try something cheaper? I'm sure Mr. Everett would prefer taking fewer meds, but he can't breathe without them."

"If he hadn't smoked for years, he might not need so many meds, Pam."

"I can't argue with that, Barb, but we have to deal with the situation we're handed. It drives me crazy that HMOs won't pay for medications to help smokers quit. I suppose they prefer paying for hospitalizations and multiple drugs later on when the patient can't breathe at all."

"S-o-r-r-y!" She spit out the word slowly so I'd get the message. "I didn't mean to get you riled so early in the morning. Your systolic blood pressure probably just rose ten points."

"You're probably right. Fine. Under justification for Mr. Everett's Accolate, write that the patient would like to breathe."

"You want me to write 'patient would like to breathe' under justification?" Barb asked incredulously.

"Yeah. Send it just like that. Let me know what they respond. If they don't reply today, call him and give him another week of samples. Thanks." Turning to Krystal, I asked, "Who's in Room 5?"

"It's your first Pap of the day. She's a fifteen-year-old sexually active teen, dragged in by her mom."

"Terrific." I took a deep breath and headed to Room 5. Believe me, it was rarely a good sign when a teenage girl was "dragged in" by her mother.

The belligerent look on the girl's face confirmed my worst suspicions. I introduced myself. "How can I help you, Angie?"

"You can get my mother off my case!" she spat out. "What I do with my life is my own affair."

"Okay, Angie. How about if I talk to your mom for a minute? Then, you and I can have a private discussion."

She nodded.

I turned my chair slightly to face Angie's mother. "Mrs. Gray, what are you hoping I can do for your daughter today?"

"I want you to check her for diseases and get her on the pill today," she shot back. "God knows what she's been doing with how many guys, but I caught her and the boy down the street in her room last night."

I looked from Angie to her mother. "Ladies, let me explain to both of you what I can and can't do today. Ma'am, without your daughter's permission, I cannot examine her for sexually transmitted diseases or obtain a Pap. That would constitute assault. If she would like to protect herself from unwanted pregnancy, I can offer her the pill following an exam, but neither you nor I can force her to take it. There are other options we can discuss, but again, she must give her consent."

"But she's only fifteen-years-old!" her mother screamed. "You have to do something!"

"She may be only fifteen, but in Colorado, she's considered an adult when dealing with problems related to birth control. What I will do is talk to your daughter alone. You may have a seat in the waiting room. I'll come get you when Angie has made her decision. I realize you have your daughter's best interests at heart, but the decisions today must be hers." And, I thought to myself, perhaps I should recommend a counselor to help these two improve communication.

After listening for several minutes to Angie's diatribe against her mom, I quietly asked, "What do you want from me today, Angie?"

"Well, I like sex, but I don't want a baby. And I don't want any disease. But I don't want my mother dictating what I'm going to do, either! And that's final!" She crossed her arms defiantly.

"Angie, I understand you're mad at your mother, and she's mad at you. That issue needs to be dealt with. Today, however, I don't care about your mother; I care about you. I care about the fact that the decisions you make now may affect the rest of your life. My job is to offer you options. I would like to offer you protection from disease and from unwanted pregnancy, but the final decisions are yours. I would much prefer dealing with these issues today rather than seeing you in a few months for counseling because you're pregnant and don't want to be."

"I'm not sleeping around," Angie replied bitterly. "My boyfriend and I have discussed the pill. I want to start them."

"Okay. I'll provide information about the pill, discuss side effects, and give you a handout. But with the initiation of sexual activity comes some responsibility. You will need an examination before I give you a prescription. If you opt to see me, you will get a full physical, not just a breast and pelvic exam. I like to make sure you have no hidden problems. You may have your exam today or you can reschedule.

"Planned Parenthood and gynecologists offer similar services, Angie, if you prefer to be seen elsewhere. If you start the pill, you will need a yearly exam. And one more thing: the pill will not protect you from sexually transmitted diseases. Condoms should also be used. Do you understand?"

"Yes."

"Would you like a few minutes to think about what you want to do, Angie?"

"No, I'd rather get my exam over with today. Does my mother have to be in here with me?"

"Not unless you want her to be."

"Then no, keep her out there."

"All right, Angie. Do I have your permission to let your mother know we will proceed with the exam today, and I will prescribe birth control pills for you as long as there are no contraindications?"

"Okay, go ahead. But no details about my exam."

"No details. I plan to obtain cultures to check for sexually transmitted diseases. You may have heard them referred to as STDs." Angie nodded. "I will call you with the results, regardless of whether they are positive or negative. But since you are considered an adult in this case, I will only give results to you, unless you give me permission to discuss results with your mother."

She shook her head.

"Fine. If you are not home, I will only leave a message that I called."

"Sounds good. But what if my mom answers and asks for results?"

"Patient confidentiality prohibits my giving her that information without your permission."

"Even if she gets mad?"

"Even if she gets mad. But I need to put in my two-cents worth, Angie, so please bear with me. I am not only a nurse practitioner, but also a mother. Although you and your mom seem pretty angry at each other, I want you to think about the fact she brought you to me today. She seems to care about you. I sincerely hope you can work out your differences, so you will feel comfortable talking to her.

"I'll talk to your mom briefly while you undress. During your exam, we'll talk. There will be no surprises. I'll explain everything I plan to do. After your physical, we'll talk more and include your mom, if you want. If not, she can cool her heels in the waiting room. I'm glad you came to see me today."

I left the room to give Angie some privacy while she changed. I pondered how I might have responded had I caught my daughter with a boy at the tender age of fifteen. I imagine I would have been furious, but hoped I would then have helped her make responsible choices. Being a parent was often no picnic.

"Pam, Room 1," Krystal announced as I completed my visit with Angie and her more composed mom. "An eight-year-old picked up a splinter in his foot. His mom can't remove it. It's been festering for three days."

A very nervous eight-year-old stared at my every move as I set up a tray with instruments.

"Bobby, you've not only got a dirty splinter in your foot, but it also has germs in it."

"How can you tell?"

"See how red it is around the splinter? And it hurts, doesn't it?"

He nodded.

"And I have to tell you that the pus oozing out is a dead giveaway."

"Oh."

"I'm going to clean your foot, take out that nasty piece of wood, and put you on medicine for a few days to kill the germs."

"Is this going to hurt?" he asked as his mom signed a consent form.

"I'm not going to lie to you. I'm going to put medicine in your foot so you won't feel me scrubbing it and taking out the splinter. It will hurt for a few seconds when I put the medicine in your foot, and then you won't feel any pain."

"You sure?" He looked worried.

"Yes, I'm sure." I turned to his mother. "Are Bobby's immunizations up to date?"

"Yes," she said.

Explaining the procedure as I went along, I cleaned the area, injected some lidocaine to numb it, and made an incision over the area where I could see the splinter imbedded under the skin. After three days of irritating my young patient's foot, the splinter fell apart. I took my time removing all the pieces. Then I cleansed the area of pus, put on some topical antibiotic and bandaged the wound. While I wrote a prescription for antibiotics, I reviewed wound cleaning and symptoms of increasing infection. A happier Bobby walked out of the procedure room.

My next patient was late, so I stood in the nursing station writing up charts. Jen, one of our medical assistants, caught my attention. "Barb told me you made up an Irish joke. She said she would have told it to me, but she can't do an Irish accent. I could use a little cheering up; my car died last night, and I don't have the money to fix it."

"It sounds like you need more than a joke to cheer you up—a few hundred bucks would probably do a better job."

"You're right. But I don't see any spare twenties floating around the nurse's station."

"We'd order a few pizzas if there was any spare cash," Barb said. "Tell her your joke, Pam. Your accent's getting better."

"Okay. But you have to understand that the Irish were not enamored of the English for a few centuries to enjoy this joke."

"Fine."

I launched into my tale. "Kathleen and Breda decide to share a couple of pints at O'Malley's Pub. They're having a bit of a laugh when one of the musicians saunters over to Kathleen and asks her if she fancies a bit of *flash*—sexual intercourse—but she waves him off. He's after pestering her all night, so she finally resorts to calling him a *fecking gobshite*, along with a few more personally aimed insults. The next morning, she feels a right *eejit* about the whole situation, so she decides to go to confession.

"So she says to the priest, 'Bless me, Father, for I have sinned. My last confession was four weeks ago.'

"Yer man gets comfortable in the confessional booth and says to Kathleen, 'And what sins do you want to confess today, my child?'

"So Kathleen leans close to the confessional screen and says very quietly, 'Father, last night, a man was after bothering me something awful and I said terrible things to him.'

134

"Father O'Reilly is surprised, because he recognizes Kathleen's voice and knows she's always been a good girl. He queries, 'What did you say, my child?'

"Kathleen takes a deep breath. 'Oh, Father, I don't think I should repeat what I said. I had a couple of pints in me at the time.'

"Father O'Reilly wants to encourage the poor lass, so he says, 'Maybe you could just whisper them in my ear, my child.'

"Thinking she could do that, Kathleen leans close to the confessional screen and whispers what she'd said into the priest's ear. Father O'Reilly pulls back, gasps, and says to her, 'Holy Mother of God! You aren't telling me you told a man to do that to himself, did you now?'

"Kathleen replies, 'That's not the all of it, Father.'

"Father O'Reilly blushes a bit, and he's glad she can't see him well through the confessional screen. 'Are you telling me there's more?'

" 'Yes, Father.'

" 'Well, my child, lean close and tell me what else you said.'

"Kathleen leans closely to the priest's ear once again and repeats the other comments she had made the night before.

"Father O'Reilly can barely contain himself. '*Jaysus*, Mary, and Joseph! I've never heard the like of it, a young one like yerself saying such things to a man.'

"Kathleen, being the good Catholic she is, starts to cry.

" 'Now, now,' yer man says. 'Don't cry. God will forgive you. It just surprises me, it does, that you would say such things to an Irishman.'

" 'Oh, he wasn't an Irishman, Father,' says she. 'Sure I would never say such things to a man of my own race.'

" 'Not an Irishman?'

" 'No, Father. He was a tourist.'

" 'You weren't saying such things to an American, were you now?' the good priest gasps. 'You know we depend on the American dollar to boost our economy, so we do.'

" 'No, Father, he wasn't an American. I've been over the moon about an American I'm dating. Sure I wouldn't say such things to an American.'

"Father O'Reilly becomes a bit exasperated. He says to Kathleen, 'Well, if you're not talking about an Irishman or an American, then what sort of man are you talking about?'

" 'Father, he was an Englishman.'

" 'Let me get this straight,' says the old priest. 'You told an English-man what he could do with himself and where he could shove...'

"Hurriedly, Kathleen cuts him off before he can finish the sentence. 'Aye, Father, he was an Englishman.'

"Letting out a deep sigh, Father O'Reilly says, 'Well, where's the sin in that? Say three Hail Marys and two Our Fathers for wasting me time.' "

Jen burst out laughing, and Krystal popped her head around the corner. "Room 5, Pam."

A tearful new mother held a three-day-old screaming baby in her arms. As I washed my hands, I studied Mrs. Sanders. It looked as though the woman hadn't slept since the birth of her daughter.

"You look exhausted, Mrs. Sanders." I touched the woman's arm. "May I hold Meghan while you tell me what's wrong?" Within seconds of her being placed in my arms, Meghan quieted.

"I don't understand why she stopped crying when you took her," Mrs. Sanders sobbed. "She's been crying for hours. She grabs onto my nipples, and they hurt so much. I'm so frustrated. I'm about ready to stop nursing. I don't know what to do."

"Is this your first baby?" I asked tenderly.

"Yes, and it's probably going to be my last. My husband's no help at all. He doesn't know what to do. My back hurts. I'm cranky. I'm so tired I can't function anymore."

"Let me try to help," I said quietly. "Meghan is already pretty smart at sensing how you feel. When I put my hand on your arm, I felt the tension. Meghan sensed that, too. You're frustrated and upset, so she's frustrated and upset. It doesn't take long for a vicious cycle to develop. She can't do anything to help herself. She just knows she's unhappy.

"You need to get comfortable. Relax your arms. When I put Meghan into your arms, cuddle her closely. If you feel tension, consciously relax. When you're nursing her, you'll have back pain if your arms are un-supported. Put a pillow or two on your lap so Meghan is brought up to your breasts instead of your bending down." I grabbed the pillow from the exam table and placed it on Mrs. Sander's lap.

"How does that feel?" I gently placed Meghan in her mother's sup-ported arms.

"Much better."

"Next, it's important to help Meghan get her mouth around the areola and not just the nipple. Let me show you how to help her nurse without hurting you." I'd glanced at Meghan's chart and had been happy to see that, despite her mom's frustration, the baby had gained several ounces since she'd left the hospital.

While Meghan nursed, I left the room to copy a handout on breast care and pick up a couple of baby books from my office. After reviewing the handout with Mrs. Sanders, I said, "One of my friends holds parenting classes for new mothers and fathers. The classes are loaded with helpful information. The local La Leche League is also a great resource for nursing mothers." I gave her both numbers. "My last concern is your lack of sleep. Do you have parents or a friend who might be willing to care for Meghan for a couple of hours in the afternoon so you can rest?"

"I have a friend who lives next door. She has three children in school and works out of her home. She offered to watch the baby whenever I need her to, but I don't want to take advantage of her kindness."

"Use her. She'll love it. You just need a few days to catch up on sleep. You can't think when you're exhausted. Please call me if you have any questions. Before you leave, you can peruse these books on baby care and development, if you don't have them already. Feel free to use this room to finish nursing Meghan. I have another examination room. Oh—one last thing. Try not to be too hard on your husband. He's probably frustrated when he sees you tired and tearful, because he doesn't know how to help. He is certainly useless as far as breast-feeding is concerned." The new mother laughed. "Do let him know how he can help you, though. Perhaps he could prepare a few simple meals or give Meghan an occasional bottle. It does get better, I promise. My three kids are teenagers and life is much easier now."

"I thought teenagers were terrible to deal with."

"The challenges are different, but at least I have five minutes to myself now and again." I touched Mrs. Sander's arm and Meghan's cheek. "I'll check on you both in a few minutes."

"Thank-you so much," Mrs. Sanders said, her eyes brimming with tears.

"You're welcome. I promise that you, Meghan, and Dad will survive this. Let me help when you need it." I quietly closed the door.

Krystal cornered me. "Pam, your next patient is late."

"This is news?" I joked.

"Since she's late, I wonder if you'd mind talking to the patient in Room 1. She made a nurse's appointment to bring in a urine sample, and she's got a whopper of an infection. She keeps getting them and wants to know why."

"Ah, the question that has puzzled women through the ages. I'll talk to her."

"Thanks, Pam. I was going to tell her to make an appointment with a provider..."

"I'll be glad to see her." I headed for my office to pull out a patient education sheet on recurrent urinary tract infections, and then I walked to Room 1.

I introduced myself to Mrs. Vaughn. "How can I help you today?"

"You could tell me why I keep getting these infections every couple of months. I'd really appreciate it."

"I have a handout on common causes of urinary tract infections, but I'd like to chat about your particular circumstances first. These kinds of infections are not uncommon in women, and usually women don't need to see a specialist, but flipping through your chart, I notice you've had five in the past nine months. That's quite a few. You have had no previous history of bladder or urine infections?"

"None. That's what so strange. I can't figure it out."

"Hmm. I notice you've had a name change as well. When did you marry?"

"Ten months ago."

"Ah hah! Now we're getting some place."

"But we lived together for two years before we married, and I never got them before. And our sex pattern hasn't changed since we married. We do it all the time...in the bedroom, under the piano, on the kitchen table..."

"I get the picture, thanks Mrs. Vaughn. Let's dig a little deeper. Have you changed the kind of soap you use to wash yourself or your clothes?"

"No, I've used the same mild soap for years. Except..."

"Yes?" I encouraged, not sure if I was ready for more enlightening comments.

"We joined a gym after we married. I don't take baths as a rule, but once in a while since we joined the gym ..."

"Maybe five times in the past nine months?"

She grinned. "Maybe. Two days ago, we played racquetball. We were pretty grimy. On the way home, we fought over who would jump in the tub first." She looked a bit sheepish. "Sometimes a bath is nice when I've had a hard workout. The warm water does wonders for my aching muscles."

It seemed to me she frequently had a hard workout: in the bedroom, under the piano, on the kitchen table... I kept my thoughts to myself, responding with just a "that's fine."

She avoided looking at me.

Oh, oh, I thought. You know that the next vision conjured up in your mind will not be G-rated when a patient avoids your eyes.

"My husband and I decided not to fight and took our bath together."

Okay, that's cool, I thought. No problem there.

"Nature being what it is, and our practically being newlyweds... You don't think having sex in the tub could have caused this, do you?"

"Some women get cystitis with increased sexual activity, but that doesn't seem to fit in this case."

"No. No increase. We do it at least once or twice a day."

"O-k-a-y..." I drew out the word. "How about the soap? What kind did you use in the tub?"

"My husband uses a deodorant soap, so we used that."

"Did you get out of the tub right after you washed?"

"Actually, no. After we, well you know, we washed each other over really well and then, well you know how nature is..." Nature in this patient's house was busier than mating season at the zoo, I thought uncharitably. "After the second time, I just laid in his arms for a while."

"And the tub was full of soap, right?"

"Yes, I guess it was."

"I imagine the soap, rather than your husband, is the culprit in this case. When you bathe, use a mild, non-deodorant, unscented soap in the bath. Wash just before you plan to get out, and don't use any bubbles or fragrance in the water. You had a physical two months ago, and Dr. Pittenger checked your kidney function. It was fine. So for now, try what I've suggested. And look over this sheet on recurrent urinary tract infections. If, in spite of making the suggested changes, you get another infection, we'll need to consider a further work-up. Okay?"

"Okay. And thanks. I feel really comfortable talking to you about this. Can I see you again?"

"If you'd like. Patients can see any of the providers in the clinic." I shook her hand and left.

My late patient had still not shown up, so I peeked in on Meghan and her Mom and then trudged down to my office to return a couple of phone calls. Two minutes later, Krystal stuck her head in the door.

"Pam, your next two patients are here. The patient that's twenty-five minutes late is so weak she can't stand up. Mrs. Andrews is an eighty-four year old patient of Dr. Hibbard's who was seen in the ER Sunday night a week ago for a staph infection. She was started on a cephalosporin antibiotic. Diarrhea began three days ago. She's really dizzy. We brought her in by wheelchair. Her appointment was made with you since Dr. Hibbard was overbooked before he even started this morning."

Based on the fact Dr. Hibbard had time to search through the wastebaskets for recyclables, he must have also had a tardy patient or two.

"I wonder if Mrs. Andrews has an overgrowth of C. difficile in her intestine thanks to the antibiotic," I said. "Cephalosporins are great drugs, but sometimes they kill so much intestinal flora that they allow resistant bacteria like C. diff to overgrow."

I scanned her medical record. "God, look at this chart! She has over twenty problems listed on her medical history list, and it looks like she's on at least a dozen medications. This is going to take some time."

"The front desk gave her a thirty-minute appointment, since you've never seen her."

"Hmm. Is anyone with her?"

"Her daughter brought her in. They're in Room 7."

"I'll be right in. I just want to check once more on Meghan and her mom. Please tell my other patient I'm running late. I'll be there as soon as possible."

"Okay."

I turned to the sink in the nurse's station. Although I always thoroughly washed my hands between patients, I washed them again before checking on Meghan and her mom. No way did I want that new baby picking up an infection in the clinic. When I entered the room, Meghan was sleeping peacefully in her mother's arms.

"She nursed on both sides," Mrs. Sanders said, beaming. "Thank-you again."

"No problem. Although it's been a long time, I still remember the day I brought home my first baby. I remember looking at her and thinking, 'If I don't kill this fragile baby in the first three months, we'll probably be all right.' "

"You were scared?"

"You betcha," I laughed. "But we survived, and in spite of me, my daughter and two sons are terrific."

Before entering Room 7, I spent a couple of minutes scanning the problem list and medication sheet. On today's progress sheet, Krystal had noted that the patient was afebrile. Krystal obtained orthostatic blood pressures while Mrs. Andrews lay on the table and then "was assisted to sitting". Her blood pressure had dropped significantly when seated, and her pulse had increased, indicating dehydration.

I flipped through the chart, reviewing the last few patient visits. Opening the door, I saw a very pale, very thin, elderly lady lying on the exam table. I walked over to her.

After introducing myself, I said, "Mrs. Andrews, you look like you're not feeling very well today." That was the understatement of the week, I thought.

Mrs. Andrews smiled wanly. "I feel too weak to sit up and it's hard to talk, because my mouth is so dry."

"She passed out in the bathroom an hour ago," her daughter interjected. "She's been so sick the last three days. I didn't know what to do."

An ambulance might have been a good choice, but I refrained from verbalizing my opinion. "I'd like to review your past medical history and your medications before examining you and ordering some fluids. You are very dehydrated. Before we start an IV, though, I need to know if you've had any problems with your lungs or heart. Have you noticed any swelling in your legs or trouble with shortness of breath? I didn't notice references to such illnesses in your chart." Mrs. Andrews shook her head.

"Mom's never had heart or lung problems other than a couple of bouts of pneumonia when she was a child."

I reviewed the problem list again. "You're a diabetic, Mrs. Andrews?"

She nodded. Her daughter spoke up. "Most of Mom's problems have come as a result of her diabetes she's had since childhood and a brain tumor that was removed about ten years ago."

Bending over my patient, I could smell the fruity odor of acetone, characteristic of very high blood sugar—diabetic ketoacidosis. "How much insulin do you take, Mrs. Andrews?" I reviewed the dosage that had been scribbled in the chart.

"Mom hasn't taken her insulin the last couple of days, because she felt too sick to eat. And she's not good about checking her sugars. I did bring a current list of all her medications, if that will help."

"That's great." I compared her list with those on the chart and reviewed the rest of the problem list with the two women. Then I began my examination. Mrs. Andrews' mouth was very dry and her lips were badly chapped. She could barely sit, but with her daughter's help, I was able to check for clear lungs. She had an accelerated heartbeat, probably secondary to dehydration. Laying her down, I examined her diffusely tender abdomen and checked for possible rectal bleeding.

"Mrs. Andrews, a short stay in the hospital will allow us to give you needed fluids and get your sugar level under control. We'll test your stool to determine what's causing the diarrhea. I need to examine you further before writing orders, but I would like to check a blood sugar right now. Additional bloods will be drawn after you're admitted. We'll transfer you by ambulance to the hospital.

"Your insulin injections will be adjusted during your hospital stay. You probably know your sugar level goes up with infection, and since you didn't take your medication the last two days, your sugar level is high. Many people with diabetes believe if they're sick and not eating much, they shouldn't take their insulin, but they should, although an adjustment in dose is necessary. And, of course, a high sugar makes your dehydration worse. We'll get you feeling better, I promise.

"Dr. Bachelder is on call today, so I will review your chart and consult with her about hospital orders. I'll let Dr. Hibbard know about your visit when he has a moment. Do you have any questions?"

"No, and thank-you. I was a little scared."

"Panic is what I've been feeling this morning," said her daughter quietly.

I left the room in search of Dr. Bachelder. She was between patients, so I shared the patient's history and reviewed orders for the hospital.

"How are you holding up this morning, Pam?" she asked.

Gloria Bachelder was really something. She was one of the most intelligent, most caring physicians with whom I'd ever worked. Each doctor had his or her own practice style. Contrary to what ran through patients' minds, there were usually several treatment options for any given illness. In our clinic, Gloria and I practiced very similarly. When I had concerns about a course of action, I often talked to her.

"I'm doing fine, Gloria. I'm just tired."

"You've been through a lot. Don't push yourself. I'd like you to go home at lunchtime. We'll keep your afternoon appointments closed this week until we see how each morning goes. All right?"

"I appreciate it. I think I'll be able to work all day tomorrow."

"Wait and see. I'll talk to Barb about calling for a medical bed for Mrs. Andrews and getting an ambulance to transport her."

"Thanks, Gloria." I popped in to see Mrs. Andrews again. Lou Ann, one of the kindest R.N.s I'd ever known, was graciously starting my patient's IV, despite her hectic day working with another provider.

...

A Pap appointment and two routine sports physicals back-to-back let me catch up after Mrs. Andrews. I'd just finished writing up the charts in the nurse's station when Krystal walked up beside me, but, unusual for her, she didn't say a word.

"Something you want to say to me, Krystal?" Her perpetual smile was absent.

"Pam, I feel uncomfortable telling you about your next patient, especially since you're going through chemotherapy."

"Spit it out, Krystal."

"Phyllis Weaver is a new patient, a sixty-eight year old woman who says she found a breast lump quite a while ago. She was afraid it might be cancer, but didn't want to know. Now she's crying in Room 7. She thinks she may have waited too long."

"Damn!" I cried out without thinking. "My apologies, ladies," I announced to the nursing staff. "Give me a minute to compose myself and I'll go in."

I willed myself to breathe. A lump rose in my throat and I swallowed with difficulty. I did *not* want to see this patient, but the physicians were totally booked. I grabbed a paper cup and gulped down water. She needs your help, Pam. She needs your help. Keep it together, woman. God, help me keep it together for her, please.

As I reached the door to the exam room, I took a deep breath. I turned the knob and walked in. Mrs. Weaver was shedding buckets of tears.

"Mrs. Weaver?" My voice cracked, and I cleared my throat. "I'm Pam Stockho, the clinic's nurse practitioner."

I sat beside Mrs. Weaver, quietly holding her hand, allowing the grieving woman time to compose herself. "I know I'm going to die," she whispered.

"Tell me why you feel that way," I encouraged quietly.

"I felt a lump in my right breast over a year ago. I thought it would go away. It didn't. I hadn't been to a doctor in five years. And then I was afraid to go. About four months ago, blood began dribbling from my nipple occasionally, and the skin of my breast darkened and puckered. My armpit is sore and there are lumps there."

"Have you noticed anything else like coughing, headaches, back pain, or chest pain?"

"Funny you should ask that. My back's been bothering me for months, but I thought it was old age. I've never smoked a day in my life, but I've developed a nagging cough the last two months. I'm also having trouble breathing, especially going up and down stairs. And the last two days I've had a fever." Krystal had noted a temperature of 103 in the chart. "That's why I decided to come in today. I thought it was just a cold, but it seems to be getting worse. And this breast lump... I figured it couldn't be anything serious because it didn't hurt. But I've read recently that cancer often does not hurt. Is that right?"

"Yes, that's right. Why don't you get undressed? I'll examine you and we can go from there. Would that be okay?" I handed her a gown.

"I have to know, doctor," Mrs. Weaver said.

"All right. I'll step out of the room while you change. And Mrs. Weaver, I'm not a doctor. I do many of the same things our doctors do, but I'm a nurse practitioner."

"I know that. But you're my doctor today, and I'm glad the appointment clerk was able to fit me in with a woman. This is difficult enough... Thanks for not giving me a lecture about waiting too long."

"I'm not into lectures unless absolutely necessary. I think you've probably been beating yourself up enough anyway. I don't need to add to your distress."

"You're right," she said. I stood outside the door and rested my head against the wall. I closed my eyes. My heart pounded in my chest. All the suppressed memories of my first reaction to the diagnosis of cancer flooded back.

After a couple of minutes, I rapped on the door. Hearing an almost inaudible, "Come in," I turned the knob.

Mrs. Weaver was sitting on the exam table. Fear filled her eyes. I gently pulled back the gown, exposing her breasts. Involuntarily, I inhaled deeply and gasped. A choking sensation suffocated me. Drops of blood seeped from Mrs. Weaver's right nipple. The whole breast looked like a rotting orange, with multiple dimpled areas, the typical *peau d'orange* of advanced breast cancer.

I felt large, tender nodes in her right axilla. Fine rales, probably indicative of pneumonia, resonated throughout the lower lobe of her left lung. Mrs. Weaver's oxygen saturation was very low—84%. No wonder she'd been so short of breath.

I obtained a medical history, completed a thorough examination, and ordered a chest X-ray. I asked Krystal to give Mrs. Weaver oxygen at 6 liters per minute through a nasal cannula. Krystal walked Mrs. Weaver down the hall and called me to the X-ray view box after developing her films.

"What's that?" she asked, pointing to a four-centimeter whitened area on the film.

"That is probably a breast cancer metastasis," I replied, despair in my voice. "See the pulmonary blood vessels on the left side? Now, compare them to the right where the cancer is—they're huge and there's evidence of new vessels. She also has a large pneumonia covering most of the left lower lobe. That's the source of her fever. Mrs. Weaver is going to have a tough time from here on. She's scared. I'll talk to Gloria, so we can get this lady admitted for her pneumonia and get a bone scan; I have an uncomfortable feeling she may have cancer in her back as well. We'll get a pulmonologist and an oncologist to see her while she's in the hospital. God, this is hard."

Krystal looked at me. "You look very pale, Pam. Are you okay?"

I turned to her. "Truthfully? No, I'm not okay. Somehow I've got to tell Mrs. Weaver the news she's been dreading for a year. And with her having waited so long, her prognosis is poor."

"Are you going to tell her that too?"

"No. Not today. It's going to be difficult enough for her to hear the word cancer. Please tell my next patient I'll be late, and then call Boulder Community Hospital and get a bed for Mrs. Weaver on the oncology ward. I need to review orders with Gloria. I'll call a report to the nursing staff and fax over orders after Gloria co-signs them."

"I don't want to darken your already deteriorating mood," Krystal said, "but your next patient is a twelve-year old rape victim."

A flash of anger shot through me. "Why is she here and not in the ER? We can't preserve a chain of evidence—nothing I collect will be admissible in court."

145

"The rape occurred over six weeks ago," Krystal responded quietly. "Her mom took her to the police only this morning to file a report. They need someone compassionate to do the exam and STD check. You were elected."

I exhaled forcefully and squeezed Krystal's shoulder. "I'm sorry for my outburst. I'm feeling emotionally overwhelmed. I'll muster up compassion, I promise." I attempted a half-hearted smile before my mood darkened once more. "Twelve! I'd cripple the SOB who took advantage of my daughter. Lord! What is wrong with this world? Give me a minute, ok, Krystal? Tell them I'll be in as soon as possible, and I'll give them all the time they need. I'm not going to rush this little girl through an exam. I may be apologizing to patients the rest of the morning, but that can't be helped."

I asked God to forgive my outburst. I received a double dose of guilt when Krystal said, "Pam, I enjoy working with you so much. I've learned a ton about caring for patients. You've often encouraged me to further my education, and I wanted you to know I've applied to nursing school. I'm thinking about becoming a nurse practitioner like you."

"You'll make a terrific nurse practitioner." And she would. Krystal had a special gift in understanding peoples' needs. I chuckled. Maybe she was complimenting me, because she sensed I needed a bit of TLC myself.

"Pam!" I heard a voice calling me from the radiology view box. "Can you look at an X-ray?"

I walked down the hall to X-ray. A picture of a minimally displaced, fractured left clavicle was illuminated on the view box. Lou Ann, our R.N. and radiology tech efficiently rolled into one, beamed at me.

"This patient walked in, so I went ahead and shot her X-ray. I thought it would be needed. I was going to put work in with Dr. Bachelder, but after talking to her, I decided you would be better suited to meet her needs. You need cheering up."

I eyed her suspiciously. Was everyone aware of my rapidly diminishing happiness reserve today? "Where is she, Lou Ann?"

"She's in Room 1. I've already laid out a clavicular strap for her. I just want you to hear her story."

I smiled but said nothing. I flipped off the view box and headed toward Room 1.

"Pam," Barb called out as I passed the nurse's station. "I just heard back from Bert Everett's HMO. They approved a six-month prescription for

146

Accolate. They apparently accepted 'wanting to breathe' as appropriate justification." She chuckled.

"Good. That's one positive thing today. I'll quickly see the lady in Room 1, finish up Mrs. Weaver's orders, and then see the twelve-year-old." Krystal had followed me into the nurse's station. "What's the young girl's name, by the way?"

"Bridget," Krystal replied.

"Bridget. Mom and Bridget must be scared to death. Please tell them I'll be with them shortly.

I opened the door to Room 1. According to the chart, I was looking at Mrs. Beech, and Mrs. Beech looked at me very sheepishly.

"Mrs. Beech, I'm Pam Stockho. I'm a nurse practitioner. I've looked at your X-ray. You've sustained a mild fracture of your collarbone that should heal nicely once we fit you with this special strap. "How did this happen?"

"My husband and I were trying a new lovemaking position, and I fell off the bed. I hit my collarbone on the nightstand."

"Ah, the old hitting the collarbone on the nightstand trick."

"Do you need further details?" she asked shyly.

"Nope, that'll do it. I think we'll leave the details between you and your husband. Okay?"

She breathed a sigh of relief. "That's fine. I appreciate it."

As I made a final adjustment of the clavicular strap and again checked the area of injury, I deadpanned, "I would seriously consider either being more careful when trying exotic positions or getting a larger bed." I left her chuckling in the room.

Krystal was waiting for me. "I looked at the rest of your schedule, Pam. After this next patient, your schedule looks pretty routine. We'll get through it. Then you can go home and rest."

"Yes, I think I do need rest. I didn't think the chemo would wear me down. It's probably the emotional component rather than the physical changes that are making me feel tired today—and grumpy. Since I saw Mrs. Weaver, I'm feeling very sorry for myself, even though my problems are nothing compared to hers. I need an attitude adjustment. Thanks for your help today, Krystal," I continued. "You've been terrific. Hopefully tomorrow I'll feel like working all day. I don't want anyone thinking I'm slacking off."

"I don't think that's been on anyone's mind, Pam. Try to enjoy your afternoon off. Tomorrow we'll make sure we get our money's worth out of you."

"Somehow I thought you might." I walked down the hall to talk with Gloria about Mrs. Weaver.

Chapter 17 - February 15th

I used stationery with the clinic's letterhead to type a note to my patients. I spent the better part of the evening composing it. It was important to let patients know what was happening to me, so they wouldn't feel abandoned while I underwent treatments. Some of my patients had become like family to me.

I paced the room, thinking about the wording of the note. It should be short and to the point—no reason belaboring the situation. I tore up several drafts before wandering upstairs and fixing a plate of cheese and crackers. I returned a couple of calls that had been left on the answering machine. I passed Bill in the family room, watching some show on WWII U-Boats.

I wandered back downstairs. I didn't want to write the letter. I didn't want to have cancer, and I didn't want to go through any more chemotherapy. I wanted to be healthy, be at work, and pretend this was a bad dream. Well, denial wouldn't solve my problem, would it? How on earth could I deny something that faced me every time I stood in front of the bathroom mirror with my bra off?

I forced myself to sit in front of the computer. I told myself I was not going to move my butt until I finished writing the note. After all, how hard could it be?

Dear friends and patients at the Family Medical Center,

Due to illness, I will be receiving treatments over the next several months that will intermittently leave me unable to care for you. I hope to be working as often as is physically possible.

Please forgive me if my periodic absences cause any problem. The wonderful doctors and staff at Family Medical Center will ensure that you continue receiving the best of care. I will be back to work full-time as soon as possible, hopefully by mid-summer.

If you feel comfortable doing so, please remember me in your prayers.

Sincerely,
Pamalla Stockho

I sat back and reread the note. In some ways I felt I *was* abandoning my patients. Continuity of care was important to me—so was teaching. I felt strongly about involving patients in their treatments, encouraging them to ask questions, giving them options, and sharing thoughts about future health plans. My nursing background provided so much of the framework for my approach to patient care. Yes, the medicine was there too, but it was the nurturing, caring, and teaching that provided the foundation of my practice and brought many back to see me.

However, there was no way I would have the energy, either physically or mentally, to worry about the outcome of tests and referrals that would transpire while I recuperated at home. So many aspects of my life were outside my control. Suddenly, I felt a crushing sense of despair and betrayal. I craved the security I had lost.

Chapter 18 - March 4th

Another three weeks passed in the blink of an eye. Facing another treatment in the morning, I'd pampered myself, putting on the gown and robe Gloria had bought for me. I'd lounged in the living room, reading *Culture Shock! Ireland* by Patricia Levy. It was light reading, but facing my next treatment in twelve hours, I'd not been in the mood for anything heavy.

I went to bed early, tossing and turning until I fell fitfully asleep. My friend, Janis, filled my dreams, probably because she'd called earlier in the evening. Janis Green and I met when we moved back to Virginia Beach in 1991. Her husband, Steve, had been loaned to the United States Navy from the Canadian Air Force—some sort of exchange program. The Greens had moved into the house across the street and quickly worked their way into our hearts.

Over a three-year period, Janis and I became close. We walked our dogs around the neighborhood—three of mine to one of hers—and commiserated on the terrible state of public schools and the deteriorating states of our mental health raising six children and two husbands between us. We shared jokes and tears and a few outings to do "serious damage" to our credit cards, which usually meant blowing a couple hundred dollars apiece.

I admitted it only once, but I felt embarrassed by how little I knew about the country bordering the United States to the North, a country comprised of only six provinces. Janis' extensive knowledge of the United States made me feel ashamed. I don't recall ever learning anything useful about Canada in high school geography lessons. I knew as much about Canada as I did about Ireland before I began studying, which was very little indeed.

In school, we'd spent loads of time studying countries that had significantly impacted the rest of the world, like England, France, Russia, and Germany. We'd pored over countries that invaded, maimed, and killed, but we'd studied little about countries trying to eke out existences in civilized fashion.

I was even more embarrassed by my lack of knowledge when I discovered, sometime after meeting Janis, that my maternal grandparents were French Canadian. I'd never known them and assumed they had emigrated from France. My mother knew little about her grandparents, and their lives in Canada, but I hoped one day to dig something up.

I had yet to visit Canada when Janis and I met, which was a shame, considering it was an English speaking country waiting to be visited without passports. Well, it was predominantly English speaking. Many fiercely proud French Canadians preferred French. My mother's grandparents had emigrated from Quebec, and they'd refused to speak English.

"Some of the *Québecois* are jerks," Janis told me, "and they will persist in speaking French to you even if you don't know the language. That is very rude, but most of the frogs are quite nice."

"Frogs?"

"Just our term for the *Québecois*," Janis informed me. "Overall, they are a very romantic people and definitely not shy about sex."

I became determined to learn more about *ze* frogs. After all, I was one of *zem* (croak).

I'd been astonished to learn that if Janis or any of her children wanted a decent job in Canada, it was imperative they master French. Canada, I was told, had two official languages, and there were French areas that wished to secede from the rest of the country. Janis' sons dutifully studied French under the tutelage of a local teacher for the three years they lived in the States.

Sometimes, I missed Janis intensely. During my dream the night before my third treatment, she commiserated with me over my bad luck in getting cancer and followed me through a day of self-indulgence. In my dream, I opened my front door to my Canadian pal.

"Are you going in *that*?" she demanded.

I looked down at the gown and robe Gloria had bought for me, and asked Janis to come in while I changed. The dream was great. I never once wondered what my friend was doing at my door, how she'd gotten to Colorado from Canada, or why I was in a nightgown in the middle of the day.

"Where are we going, Janis?" I asked, stepping into the back of a stretch limo. I'd never been in a limo, so that was a particularly cool aspect of the dream.

"Patience," she replied, a twinkle in her eye. "This is my treat. You are instructed to sit back and prepare for a wonderful day." The driver took us to a quaint little town near Boulder and parked next to What Every

Woman Deserves Spa. "We are going to have a day of pampering on me," Janis said.

The foyer was painted a pale purple. I called it purple; I'd never been any good with cute names like Elizabeth Taylor lavender or orchid mauve. Who sat around and thought up names for colors anyway? It took someone tons more creative than I was.

Healthy potted plants and trees graced every corner of the spa. Hundreds of baskets of flowers hung from the ceiling.

"I wonder who keeps their plants so healthy?" I whispered to Janis. "I should talk to their plant man. Everything I try to grow, with the exception of children and dogs, dies." At least there was a little realism in my dream.

"Good afternoon, ladies," a smiling receptionist said.

"We're here for the works," Janis informed her.

The receptionist scanned her scheduling book and checked off our names. "This way, ladies."

"How come everyone in the world is perky and good looking and I'm not?" I complained.

"Shh," Janis scolded. "Middle-aged women with three kids, a husband, and three dogs are beyond perky."

I growled at her.

Shown to a large dressing room, replete with mirrored vanities and a pink décor, Janis and I undressed and put on warm, soft blue robes.

"Do you think they have enough mirrors in this place?" I whined. "There is nothing quite like mirrors to destroy your self-esteem when you're feeling a hundred years old already."

"Will you knock this shit off?" Janis demanded. Actually, I never heard Janis curse during waking hours. She has always been much nicer than I. "You look great," she continued. "Well, pretty good for a middle-aged woman who needs an attitude adjustment."

I sneered at her. Walking through the door, we were accosted by two effusive, well-built young men. Okay, now the dream was moving in the right direction.

"This way, ladies." They massaged our upper back muscles with warm oils. Oh, yes!

"I'm in heaven, Janis."

"Pampering yourself when you go through cancer treatments encourages a positive mental outlook and boosts morale," Janis said. "I read that in a book somewhere."

These buff guys were definitely boosting my morale.

"You are not expected home for dinner, Pam. This is our day and your family is backing it 100%. By the way, Bill gave me his American Express card to use after the spa and said, 'The sky's the limit'."

Although Bill was always wonderful about my spending, I didn't think he'd ever go that far, probably because I did enough damage to our credit cards on a regular basis. But this was a dream, so I cried with happiness. The day at the spa was a lovely surprise.

"No tears, Pam. Just enjoy how this massage feels."

And I did. "Boy, these fellows really know how to use their hands." Tension was released from every kneaded muscle.

"I could almost fall asleep," Janis cooed. And she almost did.

Thoroughly relaxed, we retreated to the dressing room, showered, and put on bathing suits before heading to a whirlpool bath. Huge hanging plants and brilliant orchids embellished the room, giving further testimony to my pitiful horticultural skills. A contender for the healthiest of Pam's plants would be a pot with drooping, spindly stalks duct-taped together to keep them upright. It might boast a total of three or four blighted leaves—pathetic, but true.

The warm, swirling waters tranquilized me. "I never want to leave here," I said.

"Sorry," Janis remarked a few moments later. "We have to leave. It's time for a facial."

Under the drying cucumber-colored facial mud, I felt a slight tingling. My nose itched. Actually, it didn't itch. It felt sandpapery and damp. Something was licking my face. I woke up with a start, hardly able to breathe, thanks to two doggy paws standing on my chest. A doggy face, complete with fetid breath, hovered over my face.

"Do you have to go out, Heidi?"

Half asleep, I waited in the kitchen while Heidi sniffed around outside. After that dream, I decided to use the gift certificate to Essentials Spa that Gloria Bachelder had given me. Maybe I could convince Lisa to accompany me. Indulging my cosmetic, superficial needs might help me forget the turmoil lurking beneath.

Heidi took her time. When a meal waited, she was outside and back in a flash. But at 1:30 in the morning, when I couldn't keep my eyes open, she leisurely sniffed her way from one end of the yard to the other. She probably loved Colorado every bit as much as I did, although my heart still pined for the sea.

I grew up within a two-hour drive of Myrtle Beach, South Carolina, and I spent over twenty years following Bill from one coast to the other. I'd never lived so far from the ocean, and before moving to Colorado, my children never lived more than a few minutes from the sea. About a year ago, Gloria Bachelder mentioned she was taking Nicholas to the beach.

"Beach?" I'd questioned. "What beach could you possibly be taking him to around here?"

"Oh, we're going to the reservoir. Everyone calls it the beach."

"Maybe everyone who has never seen the sea," I'd whispered under my breath. Certainly no one who ever embraced the beauty of the Atlantic or Pacific Ocean would call the artificially placed sands surrounding a reservoir a beach. Beaches promised surf pounding shores and reed-like grasses bending in gentle breezes. They also included salty air, fish odors, and sea life decomposing at the water's edge.

Not all my memories of the ocean were pleasant, but most were memorable. In San Diego, my neighbor, Cindy, and I had taken our daughters to the beach—a day out for the girls. We hired a sitter to watch our boys. We waded into the water up to our waists, each of us clutching a small hand in ours. Without warning, an undertow grabbed us, pulling our legs out from under us. Spitting out seawater, I forced Heather out of the water over my head as I desperately tried to regain control of my legs. Cindy experienced the same feeling of powerlessness. We'd never been so scared in our lives.

Despite that incident, the sea still beckoned. Heather and the boys had spent many happy hours at rocky tide pools, collecting almost microscopic animals, algae, and seashells. While they played in tide pools near the beach, our aging golden retriever, Tigger—who succumbed to leukemia when Rob was three—regularly swam in the ocean, exercising arthritic hips. When Heather was older, she repeatedly told me she would never stay in Colorado. The sea called too forcefully.

Almost asleep again, I failed to hear Heidi at the door until she yelped, a sure sign she'd been pawing at the door for several minutes. Padding upstairs, I lay down, but sleep escaped me. My consuming thoughts were of chemo in the morning. I sighed, rose, and put on a robe. Heidi followed me, and the two of us spent the better part of the early morning watching *Defense of the Realm.*

Chapter 19 - March 5th

In spite of my dreamy day at the spa with Janis, I didn't feel like a fine looking woman as I prepared for my trip to the oncology office. In fact, I felt downright ugly and depressed. After watching *Defense of the Realm*, I'd lain in bed for nearly an hour before drifting off restlessly. I woke an hour later to the sound of Bill's irritatingly persistent alarm clock. It took twenty minutes to muster the energy to get up and take a shower.

I'd been meeting the challenge of cancer on a day-by-day basis. The tears came less frequently, but it still took little to set me off. My cauldron of bubbling emotions simmered just below the surface, and one tiny thing— something that would ordinarily be laughed off—could trigger a cascade of tears. The one bright thought for the day was that, after this treatment, I would be halfway done. Halfway—Lord, that sounded grand! I was so pleased with the thought that my mind momentarily failed to register the fact that my hands were dark brown after I rinsed soap from my hair.

I glanced down at the drain, clogged with hair, and fell apart. I wrapped myself in a towel, walked over to the bed, and wept. I was afraid to dry or comb my hair lest more fall out. I don't know how long I sat there. I let rivulets of water run down my face and shoulders, but I lacked the energy to move. Heidi jumped on the bed, put her head in my lap, and whimpered. I swear to God, if it hadn't been for that darn dog, and my feeling guilty for upsetting her, I probably would have sat there until Bill came home.

More violation. Every time I turned around, I was reminded of cancer, whether it was from clogged hair drains or burning incisional pain. I couldn't get away from it. I felt trapped and angry.

Even the darned computer did it's best to defeat me. Although I'd begun writing before my first chemo treatment, I'd stopped after less than a month. The night that had spelled the temporary end of my writing career, I'd spent an hour thinking of the perfect words, only to have a box pop up on the screen screaming *fatal error* at me. It seemed as though it were screaming at me anyway. I had no idea what I touched. I lost an hour's work. Rob tried to recover my text, but apparently it hadn't been saved to the hard drive. He said it should have occasionally automatically saved, even if, in my stupidity, I had failed to mash the save button. It hadn't.

I'd experienced such frustration at that moment that I hit the wall with the side of my hand—like that was going to help. I'd had a teen-aged boy in the clinic not long before with a similar injury, and I'd told him, "Beat up a pillow next time." To myself, I'd thought, I'm taking this wall out!

Krystal X-rayed my hand, and I'd fractured my fifth metacarpal—the bone in my hand above my fifth finger. It was not displaced, so I just wore a splint for a few weeks, but it was busted just the same. And I felt like an idiot.

Bill had said, "Nice bruise. Next time try hitting a pillow."

What I'd really wanted to do was take the computer and throw it in the trash. Until I felt ready to address the issue of my computer's irrational behavior, my writing career was on hold.

I pulled out jeans and a button-down denim shirt with sleeves that could be easily rolled up for the blood draw. I didn't tuck the shirt in. I didn't give a damn how I looked. I gingerly ran a comb through my hair, and thankfully, only a few more strands loosened. I decided to forgo make-up. Who cared anyway? I forced down some cocoa and half of an over-ripe banana.

Dr. Sitarik was quite solicitous when he saw my grim demeanor. "Your blood counts look good, Pam. Your blood counts are bouncing back pretty well between treatments. But I'm not so sure you're bouncing back emotionally."

I shrugged. "This is not my best day, doctor. I don't want to be here. I almost didn't come. I feel ugly. My hair is falling out, and I have at least a dozen mouth ulcers that have popped up in the past twenty-four hours. I don't feel like eating. My skin is turning red. I'm a freak, and I'm feeling just the teensiest bit sorry for myself today. I'm sorry."

"What you feel is normal, Pam."

I stared at him. Yeah, I thought—normal for a freak with cancer.

He continued. "No one in her right mind would look forward to these treatments. It's okay to hate them. Hate the cancer cells, too. Think about destroying them with every drop of medication that is infused."

Deep sigh. "I do, Doctor Sitarik. I do. I just want this to be over. In some ways, time has passed quickly, because I think of my life in three-week blocks now. But when I think about the side effects I'm beginning to experience, I get discouraged. I knew there would be some, but in my un-realistic mind I figured I would sail through without any trouble. Pretty pathetic, isn't it?"

"No, it's not pathetic. I hope this will be the most difficult thing you ever have to endure, and I hope the side effects will be minimal. But you're bound to have some, as you are beginning to see. Please don't get too discouraged, Pam. You can think of this as the half-full, half-empty glass. It's true you have three more treatments after today, but, on the other hand, you'll have three treatments behind you. Try to look at each day as one step closer to the end. God willing, you'll never see another cancer treatment after that."

He was right, of course. I wanted to think positively—really I did. I knew a positive attitude went a long way toward getting through any trial.

Dr. Sitarik smiled and helped me onto the table. He listened to my heart and lungs, palpated my abdomen and lymph nodes, and examined the hematoma that had developed after the blood tech nicked my antecubital vein.

"How on earth did this happen?" Dr. Sitarik asked me.

"It does look pretty gruesome," I replied. "The tech was chatting and left the tourniquet on when he removed the needle. Unfortunately, he tried to remove the tourniquet and needle at the same time. It was a bit messy."

"I noticed. I'll have a talk with him about his socializing. He's a nice guy, but he needs to pay attention instead of jabbering."

"I'll live. At least he's friendly, and that goes a long way toward easing stress in this place. I guess I'm as ready for my treatment today as I'm going to be. I don't think ice cream afterwards is going to lift my spirits."

"Go home and put on some music you like and relax, Pam."

"Thanks, doc. I will. You always make me feel better—at least I do until I walk down that hall. I'll see you in three weeks. Then I'll have gotten to the two-thirds mark."

"That's the spirit, Pam. Take one day at a time and before you know it, this will be over, and you'll only have to see my puss every three months for a check-up."

"Your puss is definitely one I wouldn't mind seeing when it's not associated with needles and nausea," I laughed.

...

Leaden-footed, I walked down the hall to the treatment station. Nodding at me, Patty encouraged me to choose a recliner. "I'll be right with you, Pam."

I had mixed feelings about being recognized. It was nice to be acknowledged, but an oncology treatment room wasn't the kind of place in which I wanted to be regarded as a regular customer. Patty seemed to be here every time I came. Didn't they give the poor woman a day off?

I chose a chair next to a middle-aged woman who looked about my age. She wore a canary yellow, floor length dress and matching turban. Her face was sallow and her head bald. The combination of jaundiced face and yellow outfit made me insensitively think of a summer squash. The woman's eyes were bright, however, and looked hopeful to me.

My IV was introduced without a problem and I hardly noticed the discomfort as the push drugs were injected. I had just opened *Pictures in My Head* when I heard a loud caterwauling coming from squash woman's companion.

I glanced over. The man was on one knee. He held a Bible in his right hand. His left hand encircled the woman's right arm. "Lord, cleanse my wife of this pestilence. Let her not suffer the indignities this disease has thrust upon her. Forgive her sins, which may have precipitated this scourge. Give us the strength to sustain her through this ordeal, oh Lord. Amen."

For pity's sake, I thought to myself. I'm as spiritual as the next man, or woman, but I couldn't see Bill or myself performing such a ritual. To intimate the woman's transgressions might have been responsible for her cancer was archaic thinking, to say the least. Actually, it pissed me off. I wasn't sure if the poor woman should be thankful for a caring husband or upset that she married an imbecile who would accuse others of bringing health problems on themselves because of misdeeds. I remembered the same ridiculous thinking when the AIDS epidemic flared in the 1970s. It amazed me that many peoples' attitudes never advanced past the days of the Spanish Inquisition and the Salem witch hunts. I tried to block out the man's loud and grating voice as he read from the Bible, but I couldn't. There would be no concentrating on my reading as long as the cacophony continued.

To my right, a large woman in black pants and a loud, orange-flowered shirt muttered under her breath. I made out the words "idiot, loud-mouthed, self-righteous, religious asshole," before smiling and closing my eyes. As one of the nurses passed by, I asked for a blanket. I drank a bottle of water and snacked on cheese and crackers while the man droned on. The thoughts I entertained about him were unkind, and I felt ashamed—just a little.

At least he was trying to help, although in a misguided way. I should have been more sympathetic, but I started giggling. I'd probably go to hell for giggling, God help me, but I found it hilarious.

When he finished, the silence was most welcome, but instead of resuming my reading, I reflected on the emotions the man stirred in me. I could have done worse than bring a Bible to read. I was acutely aware of God's existence, although I was not overly anxious to meet Him in the near future. And I imagined He understood that. I figured He was pretty amused by man (and woman) most of the time. He probably enjoyed a joke as much as anyone. Whenever I doubted His sense of humor, I took a trip to the Denver Zoo. One look at flamingoes or giraffes confirmed my suspicion that God had a lot of fun with creation. I had to believe that.

The woman dressed in orange flowers stopped muttering and fell asleep. Her head precariously flopped to one side, and she began snoring. Another couple, seated with a nurse, stared at information about chemotherapy treatments. Both looked shell-shocked. I wondered how much information either of them was absorbing. I was tired and closed my eyes. I pictured irregularly shaped cells exploding after being penetrated with toxins. The scenario had become the norm for my visits.

The battle scene slowly transformed into a bright warm day at the beach. I concentrated on relaxing my arms and legs, shifting my thinking from cells in combat to soothing sounds along a beach. I pictured myself sitting on the deck of a condo, listening to the waves, inhaling the sea air. I could almost feel a soft breeze rustling through my hair.

Pretty soon there won't be much hair to rustle through, I thought disgustedly. I opened my eyes as an old man, bent over from osteoporosis, shuffled into the room and sat down.

"Can I help you, sir?" asked one of the nurses. He flashed her a wide, toothless grin.

"Nope, just waiting to talk to Debra," he responded happily, indicating one of the nurses. "I was a victim of the vampires here about two years ago, and I'm just in to see Dr. Sitarik for a follow-up. I just wanted to remember what it felt like sitting in this chair. I'm thrilled I haven't needed one in quite a while."

"Feel free to sit there as long as you like. I'll tell Debra you're here."

I would be most grateful when I was two years cancer free. But I would be close to fifty by then, well forty-eight. There was no need to push it. Only a couple of years earlier, the thought of turning fifty had horrified me. Now, I looked at the future as years without cancer. I could live with that. Look at Sophia Loren, for goodness sake—still a goddess at over sixty. Of course, I was no Sophia Loren, heaven forbid anyone should ever get that impression, but I didn't make people want to puke, either. At least Bill loved me.

Dr. Sitarik popped his head around the corner. "How are you doing, Pam? I was worried about you. I thought I'd make sure you weren't too upset." He pulled up a chair.

Now wasn't that nice? "You are so kind, doc." He held up his hand as if to disagree with me. "No, I mean it," I continued. "I feel fortunate knowing you, although there are at least a hundred scenarios I could think of that would have suited the same purpose—and all without a hint of needles, IVs, or toxic chemicals. Seriously, I'm fine. I feel better once I'm seated back here and no longer have the option of escaping. I'm thinking of buying some cute little cotton hats to wear if more hair falls out. I think I'd like that more than a wig. And maybe people will think my skin's redness is the aftermath of some romantic cruise on the high seas. I'm okay. Thanks."

"I've noticed you don't bring anyone with you to your appointments, Pam. Most people find a friend helpful during these times."

"I know. I do bring Gabriel," I said, holding up my book. "I'm pretty introverted when it comes to my health. I find it hard making small talk when I've got poison dripping into me. I've got great friends, but I prefer discussing things other than cancer. Being here, it's hard not to think about the big C word."

He patted my hand and stood to leave. "Let me know if you need anything."

"I'll see you in three weeks. Thanks for everything." I reflected, not for the first time, that his family was very fortunate.

After he left, I eased my low spirits by reminiscing. Actually, I was particularly thankful for the memories I didn't have. Trying to hasten my aging process, my dear children had recently been sharing childhood escapades of which I had been blissfully ignorant. I always thought I was an observant mother.

I drifted off, recalling life on Mare Island. As the captain of a submarine, Bill was entitled to live in a gigantic house. It was a three-storied, white wooden monstrosity that had been divided into a duplex. Even half of the house was huge. Besides a basement and attic roomy enough for the kids to roller-skate in (much to my chagrin when I was trying to compose my thoughts), there was a pantry, large kitchen, formal and informal dining rooms, a living room and maid's quarters on the first floor.

The thought of having a maid amused me—I would have spent the whole day cleaning before she arrived. I'd hate for anyone to think me a slob. Four spacious bedrooms occupied the second floor, along with two baths. A bath and a half had been installed on the first floor as well. The pristine white, lion's footed bathtub in that downstairs bathroom was the central prop used in the continuing saga of Holly's late night skunk fiascoes and my diatribes. Mea culpa.

The old white monstrosity of a house was the one Holly tried to eat as a puppy. We sank a lot of money into repairs. Because the house was so old, having been built in the early 1900s, I invested in fire escape ladders. The children and I practiced backing out second story windows. I wouldn't have wasted my time if I had known then what I had recently learned. Off the back of the house, over the old maid's quarters on the first floor, was a flat roof. A dilapidated wooden fire escape ladder, many of the rungs missing or rotted, ran from the attic to the first floor.

Now, years later, the children had added to my ever-expanding repertoire of bedtime nightmares by admitting they frequently waited until Bill and I were asleep, then slipped out a bedroom or attic window. They scurried down the wooden ladder, which could have collapsed under any of their weights, jumped to the ground from the flat part of the roof, and rendezvoused with friends at the abandoned bomb shelters a few blocks away. Sometimes they climbed up to the roof to watch the stars. It was frightening to realize I never had a clue about their late night forages or stargazing.

While we lived in that house, Rob had suffered the only broken bone in the family. Well, other than the tuft fracture Heather sustained when Jon accidentally slammed her finger in a fire door. And of course, my recent broken finger when I fought with the wall and the wall won.

Rob was the central figure in most family injuries and mishaps. The boy was cursed, or perhaps I was cursed, because I always suffered the most agonizing chest pain when any of my children was hurt. Rob incurred almost all the lacerations in the family, but his broken arm remains among the most interesting traumatic event in the annals of Stockho family history.

Bill and I were poised to attend the annual submarine birthday ball at the officers' club on Mare Island on a balmy spring day the first year we were stationed on the island. My waist-long hair had been pulled up into a chignon and adorned with babies'-breath. I unbuttoned my blouse to slip into my gorgeous size 4, teal, low cut, sequined formal gown when the back door opened and Rob hesitantly crept in, his left arm cradling his right wrist. Did I mention it was a size 4 dress? Okay, so it was a few years ago.

"I think I broke something," he said unceremoniously.

"I think you're right," I replied, looking at the way his arm was angled just above the wrist. "It looks like you broke both bones, buddy." I fought nausea as I checked to ensure circulation to the hand was intact. I asked Bill to get some ice while I found the car keys. When I returned to the kitchen, Bill was grilling Rob about the accident.

"Sweetie, I don't think we need to worry about that at the moment," I mentioned casually, trying to sound calmer than I felt—I'd always been quite good at that. I again checked Rob's wrist and hand for good blood flow before applying ice wrapped in a dishtowel to the site. "I need to take him to the naval hospital now."

I told Bill to attend the ball without me. "You need to be there tonight, Bill. You're the commanding officer. I'm sorry I won't be able to accompany you."

"Can't you come after he gets a cast?" Bill begged.

"I don't think so, honey. This looks like he'll need surgery." I was right, and I must say I was the most beautifully coifed woman in the surgical waiting room. I am sorry to say I missed the stunt pulled by Bill and his wardroom. All the officers wore red, high-topped sneakers with their dress uniforms. Bill said the admiral was not amused.

The next day, after Rob stopped puking from the anesthesia, we went home. He insisted he had tripped over a ball, sustaining the fracture, until the attractive young lady from next-door set the record straight.

"He was trying to impress me, I think," she said. "He climbed onto the top of the clothesline and held his arms out saying, 'Look at me, I can fly.'" Rob denied it, and still does, but I saw the truth in his beady little eyes. Mothers know these things.

All in all, the kids hadn't gotten into too much trouble over the years— at least, not much I knew about. I hoped they didn't have any more historical surprises for me. My aging heart couldn't take much more.

Bill enjoyed his share of fun as well. And no, they didn't involve women; despite his allusions to games and dames on numerous shore leaves, he knew what would happen if he ever brought me home a little gift from his overseas excursions. In the movie, *Ruthless People*, Bette Midler simulated grabbing a pair of testicles and snipping them off with a pair of scissors before throwing them over her shoulder. Bill saw the movie with me, and believe me, my making that little Bette Midler gesture was enough to make him reach down and protect his gonads. Nope, we never had problems in that department.

He enjoyed his tour at Mare Island Naval Shipyard, but he especially enjoyed the sub's transit from California to its homeport of Charleston, South Carolina, after the boat's overhaul was complete. Going through the Panama Canal, the troops enjoyed a cookout on a Weber barbecue grill, which was placed on the turtleback, or deck, of the sub. There had also been opportunities for skinny-dipping during the trip. A number of sailors sustained sunburns in areas rarely, if ever, exposed to the sun. I heard that sitting down and urinating presented a challenge for several days. No pictures that I know of made it home to the wives.

I woke up chuckling. I looked up at my IV, now empty. Blood backed up into the tubing. Debra walked by, pulled out the IV catheter, and I was free for another three weeks. I drove home, made dinner, and went to bed.

Chapter 20 - March 13th

Although I couldn't say I remembered many dreams from years past, those I experienced during chemotherapy seemed especially vivid. Perhaps brain cells under siege from chemo became a little brighter before they burnt out, much like a supernova. The intensity of dreams with an Irish theme might also have been due to my developing love for the Irish people. I greedily studied their history, culture, poets, and authors. For the first week after each chemo treatment, I watched too many movies, but when I felt better, I read voraciously.

I fell asleep reading *Ireland: Its Myths and Legends* by Kay Retzlaff, and I was soon adrift in a small boat that landed on a verdant shore near a thatch-roofed pub. A tall, dark-haired man guided me by the arm into the dimly lit bar. Low wattage bulbs extended from the brass arms of slowly rotating ceiling fans. The interior décor was subdued, with mahogany paneling running halfway up the wall. Above that, flocked green wallpaper served as a backdrop for Irish coats of arms. The beautiful bay windows of the tavern depicted scenes reminiscent of the *Book of Kells*, a historical illuminated manuscript of the Four Gospels. A magnificent marble statue of the epic hero of Irish folklore, *CúChulainn*, stood prominently on a pedestal in a lighted corner near the bar.

"They probably stood him in the corner so drunken sods wouldn't knock him over. What a shame that would be," my companion said, in a decidedly Irish accent—County Dublin I thought. I didn't recognize the man, but his salt-and-pepper hair framed a handsome face that reminded me of dreamy Gregory Peck, and his steel-blue eyes danced. The corner of his mouth curled into a half-smile as he spoke. He strained to seek his friends in the crowded pub.

"Kevin!" someone shouted from the farthest corner of the pub. The man, now named, nodded in the direction of the voice, grabbed my hand, and guided me past the marble-topped bar to the table from which the voice emanated. As we approached, we were regaled with the sounds of bawdy songs and raucous laughter. I stopped momentarily in my tracks, but Kevin encouraged me.

"Come on. They're just letting off a bit of steam. I promise to put in a good word for you if the *guards* show up."

"*Guards?*"

"Police."

Approaching the table, a voice in the dark called out, "If it isn't yer man coming at us. Kevin, who's your new *mot*?"

"What's a *mot*?" I asked as Kevin pulled out a chair for me.

"A *mot* is a girlfriend." Kevin beamed. "Good evening, gentlemen. And I do use the term loosely."

"*Wisha*! Be nice tonight, Kevin, or you'll find yourself waking up dead in the hospital."

"Before you say things you may regret for the rest of your miserable life, ya *hoor*, I'd like to introduce you to my friend, Pam," Kevin replied.

Mumbled "Howya?" and "*Dia Duit*"—hello—filled my ear.

Kevin continued. "You may recognize Liam here, Pam—he's been in a few popular films. He seems to make the ladies' hearts pound." Okay, not Gabriel Byrne, but Liam Neeson got my attention as well.

"Michael's the one over at the bar buying a bottle of Irish whiskey. Hey, Michael," Kevin shouted, "say hi to Pam." Michael doffed his hat and bowed. He paid for his bottle and walked back to the table.

"The one with the big mouth here, Seán, was a friend for years before he ruined a perfectly good relationship by marrying one of my sisters. We've been through some tough times together, haven't we, Seán?"

"We have," said Seán, sipping his porter. "We've been on the crawl in Dublin more times than I can count, drowning our sorrows in pints of Guinness. Of course, that was before I married." He sighed. "For old times sake, let me stand you and your lady friend a round."

"Fine," Kevin answered, sitting down, "and I'll stand the next round. Bring a half-pint of plain for Pam and a pint for meself."

When Seán returned to the table, Kevin asked, "How is Brigid, Seán? I haven't seen her in weeks."

"The night before I left Dublin, she was wailing like a banshee."

"Why?" asked Kevin. "What did you do this time?"

"Nothing," Seán protested. "I had in mind to meet up with the lads for a couple of pints before flying to the States. That's the all of it. It was a shameful sight her scolding me in front of the neighbors."

"Did you go then or stay home with your wife?" I asked, not realizing until a moment later what an ignorant comment that was to make.

"Did I go? Did I go? What kinda fool question is that? Of course I went! I knew I wouldn't be home for two months. But terrible put out, she was. 'Don't make me lose my temper,' says she. I got home late, and she turned her back to me in bed. I'm hoping she'll forgive me by the time I get home."

"That's what you get for marrying," Kevin laughed. "Women are always trying to keep a man from doing what comes naturally."

Their laughter almost kept me from hearing the phone. I picked it up. "Pam, is that you? Were you sleeping?"

"I guess I was, Mom. I seem to spend most of my waking hours dodging sleep. How are you?" I could tell from the care packages Mom had recently sent, including letters, grocery coupons, magazine articles, and cartoons, that she had been more worried about me than she'd let on during our frequent phone conversations.

"I'm fine, but more to the point, how are you, Pam?"

"I've had three treatments, so I'm half-way home. It's something to celebrate. Bill is taking the kids and me out to dinner in LoDo this afternoon. We're going to a restaurant I've been dying to try."

"Which one?"

"Dick's Last Resort."

"Dick's Last Resort? Isn't there a similar restaurant in Myrtle Beach?"

"Yes, it's the same chain."

"Didn't they put a condom hat on Heather's head and insult her all evening when she went with a friend?"

"That's the place," I said. "It helps to have a good sense of humor to eat there. If you take offense at the waiter's abrasive manner, you won't have any fun at all. They're encouraged to be a bit nasty so patrons feel they're getting their money's worth."

"And you want to eat there?" Mom asked, surprised.

"I do, believe it or not."

"You don't take after me in that department. How's the writing coming along?"

"I'm on hiatus at the moment. My computer and I had a serious difference of opinion. The computer won. And so did the wall."

"The wall?"

"Yup. It's a long story. I've been doing a lot of reading when I'm not too ill."

"Anything I'd be interested in?"

"I'm reading Irish humorists at the moment: J. P. Donleavy, Brendan O'Carroll, and Roddy Doyle. I needed a break from James Joyce. I can only take so much heavy reading. When I read Joyce, I feel like I haven't got a single functioning brain cell."

"How about sending me a couple of books when you're finished with them, Pam? I could use a few laughs."

"I'll do that, Mom. Have you been over to Linda's lately?"

"I've been going over Wednesdays to stay with Maggie while Linda and David bowl."

"That's nice of you. How is Maggie?"

"She's great," said Mom. "I let her run through the woods whenever it's nice. One of these days she'll catch a squirrel. She loves running after them."

"I hope she doesn't catch anything. Yuck! Linda's so lucky to have a home in the woods. We have open spaces where the dogs can run, but it's a drive to get there."

"Maggie is more than a dog, Pam. She's Linda's baby."

"I know—and your granddog."

"You're sure you're okay, Pam?"

"Yeah, I'm fine. Really."

"I wish I could come help you."

"I've got all the help I need. Thanks. You've got enough to do getting back on your feet after bilateral hip replacements. Don't worry about me."

"That's what mothers do."

"Don't I know it? I'm going to come out to visit for a couple of weeks after I finish my treatments. How does that sound?"

"It sounds great. We'll pamper you while you're here."

"I'll look forward to it." The front door slammed.

"Mom? Are you here?" Heather called.

"Upstairs, Heather… I'd better go, Mom. Heather's here, so I need to get ready for Dick's."

"Have fun! Talk to you later. Love you."

"I love you too. Bye."

Heather walked in with a glorious floral arrangement she'd picked up from William at the Louisville Florist. The man, with help from Shelley, who was an artist in her own right, created magical bouquets. Heather frequently showered me with flowers at home and work, for no other reason than to let me know she was thinking of me. A card attached to a recent bouquet that arrived at the Family Medical Center had read: "World's

Greatest Nurse Practitioner". I casually left that card on my desk for days. The one that read: "World's Best Mom" was in put in my keepsake box.

"The flowers are gorgeous, Heather. Thank-you so much!"

"You're welcome, Mom. I just wanted you to know I appreciate all you do for me."

What a wonderful kid!

...

We piled into Bill's jeep for the twenty-five minute trip to Denver. He'd loaded his CD player with Irish music.

"Dad, don't you have anything but Irish music?" Heather wailed. "That's all Mom listens to these days."

"That's not all I listen to," I challenged.

"It sure seems like it," she grumbled.

I reached over and turned off the CD player. "We could just talk," I suggested, so we spent almost half an hour catching up on school news, boyfriends and girlfriends, and future plans. That wasn't as easy as it sounds; pulling information out of the kids when they hadn't initiated the conversation was like dragging them to the dentist, with my asking questions and their replying in short sentences sure to prevent imparting much information.

"Fine." "It's okay." "We talked about that last week, Mom." Not exactly riveting dialogue, but it passed the time.

Dick's would be packed later in the evening, so we had decided to go early. The five of us found a relatively empty restaurant when we arrived.

"Well, what do you want?" snapped a less than nattily dressed young man at the door. Besides holes in his shoes and blue jeans, he sported a T-shirt that read, *I Got Crabs at Dick's.*

"We would like a table," Bill responded.

The young man motioned toward the large dining room. "There doesn't seem to be a lack of selection. I think you're big enough to find your own table. Pick out something that suits you."

"I think I'll use the ladies' room first," I said.

"Would you like me to broadcast that on the intercom?" the young man inquired, hand on his hip.

"I'll pass on that, thanks. Could you point the way, please?"

"If you would open your baby blues, you would see the yellow neon sign flashing, *2 P* to your right," he responded testily. "Follow that down the stairs. You shouldn't have any trouble. The men's room has a sign on it that says *Little Dicks*. That's not the one for you. That is, unless there's something you aren't sharing about yourself."

I found the ladies' room at the bottom of the stairs. After washing my hands, I spent a couple of minutes inspecting the condom vending machine next to the sink—such an interesting selection of colors. Making my way up the stairs, I was accosted by an irate waiter.

"Your significant other and the monsters have already given me their orders. It would be appreciated if you would have a seat and decide what you want so I can serve you and get you out of here. What do you want to drink?"

"Do you have Guinness?" I asked, trying to act cool.

"Is this some kind of conspiracy?" the waiter demanded. "I just got the third degree from your pal for not having Guinness available. We happen to like Murphy's stout better. I'm sure your unrefined palate won't be able to tell the difference. Your friend thinks otherwise. He must figure himself to be a man of the world. Humph!"

"I'll try a pint of Murphy's," I laughed. "You guys are a riot."

"Oh, the little lady thinks we're here for her amusement. Well, pull up a seat at the table with lover boy and look at the menu. I'll give you three minutes and thirty seconds to make your decision or I'll make it for you."

I tried unsuccessfully to suppress a laugh as I walked to the table. My mouth hurt from grinning. I looked at rows of tables that looked like they'd been rescued from a junkyard. The chairs were old and mismatched, some of them with only shreds of tattered fabric clinging to the frames. It was to one of these that the waiter motioned me.

"I can't sit on that!" I exclaimed. "My butt will fall through."

"Such language from a supposed lady," replied the waiter, feigning astonishment. "I presume you are known to curse on occasion, too."

"On rare occasions, when it's warranted."

"And you obviously drink, too, judging from your beverage order," he stated pointedly.

"Once in a while."

"Are all three of these your children?" he asked.

"Yes." I wondered where his line of questioning was going.

"Well, aren't you a fine example for them!" he concluded haughtily. "Now, as far as your precious derriere is concerned, just straddle the chair. Most broads your age are pretty good at straddling things, now aren't they?"

I chose another seat. Bill was practically rolling on the floor. His laughter echoed through the restaurant.

"These fellows are great, Mom," Rob said. I silently prayed this was one job he wouldn't consider for a career.

The waiter returned with pieces of white paper, which he threw at us, followed by sets of utensils wrapped in torn pieces of material. He tossed a menu at me.

"Three minutes and thirty seconds to make your decision," he declared. "I'll be back."

"He sounds like Arnold Schwarzenegger with that, 'I'll be back'. I'm shaking in my boots," I whispered.

"I have a gift for the smart-mouthed lady," the waiter divulged a few minutes later. He held a paper hat formed in the shape of a condom. On it in red letters, he had written, "I drink booze. I swear like a sailor...I'm a fine example for my children". He placed the hat on my head.

"Do I have to wear this condom hat during dinner?"

"Only if you want to make your waiter happy," he replied, looking at me darkly. "And if I were you, I wouldn't want to make your waiter unhappy. What do you desire to fill your big mouth with?"

"I'd like to order one of your sandwiches listed under *Road Kill on a Bun*," I told him.

"Well, which one?" he demanded. "Or do I have to consult my crystal ball to figure it out?"

Order in hand, he huffed and walked away. Looking at a line of T-shirts hung from the ceiling, I asked another waiter, "Are those shirts for sale?"

"No," he retorted. "We just hang them there with prices listed so idiots like you can ask if they're for sale. Of course they're for sale if you can cough up the dough. Talk to your waiter."

Sipping our pints of Murphy's Stout—Bill and I, not the kids—we looked over the T-shirt selections. Heather chose one that read, *Contrary to Rumor, Real Women Love...DICK'S...Last Resort.* Jon bought one emblazoned with, *I Don't Know Jack, but I Know Dick,* and last but not least, Rob picked one like the less than nattily dressed greeter wore, which said, *I*

Got Crabs at Dick's. The mother in me pined for lost innocence, but I'll admit I'd been as big a contributor to that as anyone had.

Our waiter threw plates of food in our general direction, and we ate in relative silence. Amazing! At home, I couldn't get them to behave at the table, but at Dick's, when we had a waiter who made our table comments look positively tame by comparison, the kids were on their best behavior. Maybe they realized they couldn't compete with this pro, or maybe they were worried I'd want to continue the talks we'd started in the car.

Chapter 21 - March 27th

I always loved the hope for new beginnings that spring brought. I craved hope. I'd been keenly aware of the beginning of life during the drive into Boulder for my fourth chemotherapy treatment the day before. Boulder cattle herds had thinned appreciably during the past couple of weeks, but driving on, I found the missing cows. They'd been placed in a separate pasture, each one hovering near a calf.

I thought about those calves while I waited for the IV to drip in during chemotherapy. No new characters presented themselves as I quietly sat and read. I desperately wanted to be done with the place. I so admired the nursing staff, especially Patty, whose smile cheered those of us who regularly haunted the treatment room. I had to admit my frame of mind improved once the IV was in and the drugs started—another step closer to the end. The fear of death was no longer foremost in my thoughts, although it took little to pop the thought into my head when my guard was down.

After chemo, I drove home and spent the day with Gabriel Byrne and Harrison Ford, sipping ginger ale until nausea hit. I dragged myself to bed, waking early this Saturday morning to birds chirping at my window. Truthfully, as romantic as that sounds, I actually heard the birds after I woke. It was Bill's snoring that forced my eyes open. Moaning, I considered pulling the covers over my head, but the dogs' insistence and Bill's annoying opus got my rear moving.

I wandered outside to drink in the smell of freshly mown grass. I stood on the deck savoring daffodils and crocuses, while the dogs killed grass with their urine. Buds dressed the trees, which convinced me we'd endure another snowstorm before long, ensuring broken branches weighted with wet spring snow.

While I waited for the dogs, I stretched out in a chair, hiked up my nightgown, and enjoyed the warmth on my legs. The thermometer didn't register forty degrees at that point, but I experienced a hot flash, a new sensation thanks to the chemo, and I had all I could do to keep from ripping my gown off. The thought of being arrested for indecent exposure didn't worry me as much as scaring my neighbors, so I restrained myself.

Heidi and Holly padded up the stairs and lay at my feet. Heidi rolled onto her back and fell asleep. Her intermittent snoring intruded upon my tranquility. Probably another trick she'd learned from Bill, although she was not as loud as he. I stared at Heidi's spread-eagled position and couldn't help laughing.

"Ladies do not lay like that, Heidi." I reached over and gave the dog's belly a scratch. Holly, always quick to notice my willingness to dispense affection, got up and lumbered to my other side, nuzzling my hand with her muzzle. I petted her head. It felt great to be needed. The dogs placed me on a pedestal, no matter how little I deserved the adoration and devotion.

It could have been adoration or it might have been hope I'd let them get away with ignoring everything I'd taught them. Every spring, I spent weeks re-training the dogs to relieve themselves on the grassy patch at the far side of the house, but every winter they reverted to doing their business as close to the house as possible, partly due to the cold and partly due to the occasional one to two feet of snow they were required to trudge through. Heidi frequently didn't even make it off the back deck, squatting right outside the door. Scolded, Heidi would stare at me as much as to say, "You're kidding, right? You don't really expect me to trot my eight inch legs through two feet of snow just so you can avoid cleaning the deck, do you? Okay, I'll do it if you will." And she'd complete her business giving me a dirty look.

Hannah rolled back and forth across the greening grass. Watch where you roll, girl, I begged silently, remembering I'd had every intention of scooping up the poop a couple of days before.

A gentle breeze relieved the hot flash, and the wind chimes on the corner of the house tinkled melodiously. How could my morning be any better than this? I opened a folder on my lap, a folder prepared for me by Lisa and other clinic accomplices. Trying to cheer me up, they'd collaborated on the first chapter of a cheesy detective novel, detailing the P.I. exploits of one Panama Stockholm. Lisa and her cohorts had spun a yarn based on my daring, but highly fictionalized, exploits in the crime-ridden capital city of Colorado. I was deeply touched.

The name, Panama Stockholm, had not been pulled out of the air. On no fewer than three reports I'd received from specialists' offices to whom I'd sent patients, I was listed as Dr. Panama Stockholm. Lisa and I frequently joked about the alias, and I'd commented I'd considered using the moniker to lead a double life. I could dress in any of the many holiday outfits for which I'd become infamous in the clinic—St. Patrick's Day Leprechaun, Easter bunny, Fourth of July flag salesman, Halloween witch/ghost/pumpkin or Christmas Santa/snowman/reindeer. I had worn appropriate attire close to each holiday for the amusement of young patients for years, but I'd been such a hit that I expanded the holiday garb to several weeks before any festive day arrived. I cut back only when Dr. Hibbard commented that it was "a little early" for any particular outfit.

A post-it note attached to the folder captured my immediate attention. "By day, Pamalla Stockho is everything a noble nurse practitioner and mother should be...but at night, Panama Stockholm, private eye, takes to the underbelly of Denver's sleazier districts, ferreting out the frightening truths behind the lies of clients and prey alike..."

Here for the first time are excerpts from Lisa and her gang's work. She's going to kill me for sure!

The Adventures of Panama Stockholm

Panama Stockholm breathed a sigh of relief as she pulled off her Halloween themed smock and pumpkin earrings. God! She wondered. How did Pam Stockho stand her sweet and orderly world? Pulling on a black fedora and one skull and crossbones earring, she revved up her Harley and headed for a bar in Five Points, in downtown Denver. Rumor had it she'd find a one-eyed man called Golden-eye at the White Front on Colfax. She'd been looking for him for a long time.

Her mind wandered back to all the grimy, sleazy, low-down bars she'd haunted the last few months in pursuit of Golden-eye. A half-smile pulled at the corner of her mouth. It hadn't been a bad month at all. Any woman who bathed at least once a week could get her drinks for free in Five Points, and Panama made sure she kept her appointment with the tub every Thursday.

Panama's informant, Dickey Fingers, said there were two low-life sleazes named Golden-eye, but the one guilty of the heinous crime she had been hired to solve could be either. Not until she questioned each would she know which was her man.

She ordered another shot of whiskey. All at once a guy came through the doors as though he had been tossed in. Under the dirt and greasy hair, she could detect he had a glass eye, a gold one at that.

"What's your real name?" she demanded.

He sneered at her. "How about buying me a snort, Toots?" He leered suggestively at her fishnet-clad thighs. Always one to oblige,

Panama hiked her black leather skirt several inches higher and, holding her breath, leaned suggestively toward her prey.

"Tell me your name and I'll buy you a whole bottle of this transmission fluid, big boy." Her voice was a low, seductive purr, but the steel in her eyes belied the accommodating appearance.

"Who wants to know?" He belched the question.

She reached for his neck and pinned him against the bar.

"No offense meant, honest, lady! Billy Geronimo's the name my sire fastened on me more years ago than I can remember." Golden-eye continued to shrink before Panama's cold appraisal.

Hiding her disappointment, Panama slid off her bar seat and sauntered suggestively toward the exit, fully aware every male eye in the bar that could focus was watching her leave. So, not *her* Golden-eye. She'd never heard of Billy Geronimo.

It was nearly three in the morning when Panama eased her Harley Fat Boy into her driveway and cut the engine. It wouldn't do to wake Heather, Jon, or Rob, who might question her late night activities. Kids these days! They seemed to think they had a say in her every move!

She only had time for two and a half hours sleep before she was due at the clinic. She understood very well that her own health would suffer if she continued to burn the candle at both ends.

At the end of the day, she ducked out without finishing her patient charts. She wanted to get the family fed and get to the Glory Bar to seek Golden-eye again. Tonight she was wearing full leathers and Harley replica earrings. Hours went by and still no sign of him. Could someone have tipped him off? It was almost two a.m. before she saw him slink in the door.

The name Golden-eye suited him—he had a yellow star tattooed over his left eye. The Harley Eagle tattooed on his shirtless chest excited Panama. His unzipped leather vest allowed her to appreciate the artist's work, which was complimented by a thick mat of glorious brown hair. Tattooed snakes encircled the bulging muscles of both arms.

He sneered contemptuously. She shivered. She'd come unarmed, and that was unsafe—not even a syringe with a 20-gauge needle in her handbag. But she'd finally seen him—her Golden-eye. She'd be ready next time, but it was time to head home and get some rest.

On the way home from the Glory Bar, Panama was forced to detour through a construction site. She ended up lost on a dark and empty street. Her bike broke down in the middle of nowhere. Getting off her hog, she heard a rustling noise.

Before she could react, a shadowy figure appeared. He wore a bandana over long braided hair. It was too dark to see the yellow star tattoo she knew was over his left eye, but she could see the Harley Eagle gleaming through his luxuriant mat of chest hair, thanks to the single street light that flickered on and off. The full moon illuminated the silver toes of his cowboy boots.

Panama ran her eyes slowly over his form, lingering over his washboard abs and the ample bulge in his jeans.

"You would have to be a crook," she sighed with disappointment. "I'm going to have to take you in, you know."

"Whatever you say, Ms. Stockholm." He smiled slightly and flicked open the first button on his skin-tight Levis.

"Oh, hell!" She took a step toward him and shrugged out of her black leather jacket. "No one ever said *when* I gotta bring you in." She shoved him down on a pile of construction debris and...

End of Chapter 1

What a great bunch of gals! They'd made my day. A smile was plastered on my face, just as it was whenever Dad called with another lascivious joke. After an Army career of over twenty years, Dad worked oversees for the State Department's Agency for International Development. He worked in Vietnam, Egypt, and Pakistan before retiring to Myrtle Beach, South Carolina. Until I married a military man, I never appreciated how hard it must have been on Mom, raising two daughters during the years Dad had been gone for up to a year at a time.

Although Dad had chugged down more than his share of booze, his health improved after he joined AA and started working out at a local gym. At seventy-six years of age, he was in better shape than he'd been at forty. He spent the better part of his days on the golf course when he wasn't mapping out trips to military conventions that were held around the country.

I eased my weary, aching body out of my chair and headed inside, bound for the kitchen to make blueberry muffins for breakfast. Bill worked long hours during the week, so I invariably beat him out of bed weekend mornings. The kids were rarely up before noon. I threw the muffins in the oven, showered, dressed, tossed a load of laundry into the washing machine, and was about ready to sit down for a rest when the phone rang.

"Stockhos. Good morning."

"Morning beautiful," the cheerful voice responded.

"Dad! It's great to hear your voice. I was just thinking about you. How are you?"

"I'm fine, Pam. How are you doing?"

"Tired, but otherwise okay. I had my fourth treatment yesterday. I still have my hair, although it has really thinned, and I've only gained a couple more pounds."

"Glad to hear it. You said you were thinking about me. Anything in particular?"

"I was thinking about what great shape you're in since you exercise so much. How's your golf game? Still playing every day?"

"Just about."

"Do you recall when I asked you that question a few years ago, and you said you hadn't been playing much?"

"I remember. That was before my first angioplasty—would have been the end of 1990."

"Yes. You were experiencing chest pressure after the first nine holes."

"I figured I was just getting old—all that huffing and puffing. Glad I listened to you about seeing my doctor. A little roto-rooter work did wonders. I've been great ever since."

"Good! You won't ignore those symptoms again, will you?"

"Nope. I promise."

"I have a joke for you, Dad."

"Okay, I'm ready. Where'd you hear it?"

"Someone sent it to me on the Internet—it's been circulating in recycle-conscious Boulder."

"Okay."

"A Texan, a Californian, and a Boulderite are chugging their beverages of choice when the Texan empties a bottle of tequila, throws it into the air, pulls out a gun, shoots the bottle, and sprays glass shards over everyone in the bar.

" 'Hey!' someone exclaims. 'What did you do that for?'

" 'I'm from Texas,' declares the Texan. 'We've got plenty of bottles of tequila down there.' He returns to guzzling tequila.

"After a few minutes, the Californian empties a bottle of wine, throws it into the air, pulls out a gun, shoots the bottle, and sprays glass over everyone in the bar.

" 'Hey!' someone hollers. 'What did you do that for?'

" 'I'm from the Sonoma Valley,' declares the Californian. 'We've got plenty of bottles of wine where I come from.' He returns to drinking wine.

"A few minutes later, the Boulderite puts down his guitar, places his empty bottle of Fat Tire on the bar, shakes his long hair out of his eyes, adjusts his Birkenstocks, and pulls out a gun. He throws his bottle into the air, shoots the Texan and the Californian, and deftly catches his empty bottle before it hits the floor.

" 'Whoa!' screams a bar patron. 'What did you shoot those two fellas for?'

" 'I'm from Boulder. We've got too many Texans moving in here, and too damn many Californians. But bottles—those you can recycle!' "

Dad laughed, and it was good to hear. "Okay, Pam, I've got one for you."

"Ready."

"Two English women, Margaret and Elizabeth, spend half an hour swimming in the ocean. Shivering, they run up to the beach and grab their towels, laughing while they dry off. Margaret reaches into the top of her bathing suit, pulls out a cigarette and lighter, and lights up.

"Elizabeth stares at Margaret, and exclaims, 'How did you keep your ciggies dry, then?'

" 'Easy,' replies Margaret. 'I went to the chemist and bought a pack of rubbers. I slipped the ciggies inside, along with me lighter, and they've stayed nice and dry.'

" 'I'll have to get me some,' replies Elizabeth. The next day, Elizabeth walks down to the drug store and asks for a package of condoms.

" 'What size?' inquires the sales clerk.

" 'Oh, about the size to fit a Camel,' Elizabeth replies."

"Not bad, Dad. Not bad at all."

"At least your spirits are good, Pam. Keep a positive attitude. I know you'll whip this thing."

"Thanks, Dad. It's been good talking to you. I hear Bill making noises upstairs. I think I'll slip into bed for a nap. I have little physical reserve the first few days after chemo. "

While Bill showered, I slipped into bed and pulled the covers up to my chin. Minutes later, he loomed over me, a towel around his waist.

"Mind if I hold you for a few minutes?" he asked, slipping into bed.

"You may, but *can* you just hold me?" I laughed.

"I had an exhausting week at work. I'm too tired to do anything else," he said.

"Isn't that supposed to be my line?" I teased.

"Please don't let anything happen to you, Pam. I couldn't bear to live without you."

"Only the good die young, my dear. I'll live forever." As I cuddled against him, I felt what I presumed was not a gun in his pocket.

"If the good die young, you would have died long ago, Pam."

"I knew you wouldn't be able to just hold me, Bill."

He pulled me closer. "I guess I'm not that tired."

Chapter 22 - March 30th

Blessed lunchtime followed a very busy morning in the clinic. A drug rep cornered me outside the kitchen.

"This calculator will determine a woman's risk of developing breast cancer over her lifetime," the rep told me. "It's called the Gail Model Risk Assessment Tool. You enter her statistics, and you can determine if the risk is high enough to warrant prophylactic tamoxifen to help prevent cancer. I don't have any patient charts with me, but let's make up some statistics, so I can show you how to use this."

"How about using me as an example?" I asked, knowing I was setting up the poor woman. Unfair of me, and not like me usually, but I was tired of hearing/talking/thinking about cancer—like it would all go away if no one mentioned it.

"Okay, we can try that. We'll put in race here as white. Age?"

"46."

"Age at menarche and age of first childbirth?"

"10 and 24."

"Number of female relatives with a history of breast cancer?"

"None."

"Number of breast biopsies and whether they were benign or suspicious or cancerous?"

"One and it was benign—a fibroid adenoma."

"Well, your risk will be quite low, and the calculator agrees with me. Isn't it great how easy that was?"

"I love statistics," I remarked, uncharitably. "By the way, I was diagnosed with breast cancer in December."

The rep's face fell. "I'm sorry to hear that, Pam. But this is a valuable tool to assess the risk of patients who have a family history of breast cancer. Prophylactic use of tamoxifen can significantly decrease the risk of developing familial breast cancer."

"I know, and I'll use the tool. It will be helpful to give women an opportunity to evaluate their risk and weigh the benefits of using the drug versus the dangers of possible side effects."

The drug rep fidgeted. I was making her uncomfortable, and that wasn't fair. She wasn't responsible for my cancer, and tamoxifen helped many. I knew that. I could think of one word to sum up my attitude at that moment, and it was BITCH. Not hearing about cancer in my line of business was impossible, but while I fought my own battle, I wanted to pull myself into a protective cocoon and avoid the word and the disease.

Mentally berating myself, I mustered a smile for the woman. "I'm sorry. Sometimes hearing the word cancer makes me moody. I promise to be good."

She nodded, and we reviewed potential side effects of the drug—side effects I might have to deal with in a few months.

As I took my cooled-off lunch to my office, I almost ran into Gail. She was a fabulous head nurse, always concerned about those who worked with her.

"Feeling confrontational today?" she asked smiling. "I heard your discourse with the drug rep."

"It was not my best display of behavior. I'm hungry and I'm tired of hearing about breast cancer."

"I know it's difficult," Gail sympathized. "By the way, staff and patients are commenting about how lovely you look in that gorgeous outfit you have on today."

"Thanks. I wish I felt lovely. It's funny, but every time someone comments on how nice I look since I lost weight, I want to say, 'I've got breast cancer—it must agree with me.' "

"Goodness! Is there anything I can do to brighten your day, Pam?"

"No. I'm okay. It's been a long morning, I'm exhausted, and I'm not looking forward to working this afternoon. How about asking the front desk not to give me any laceration repairs this afternoon. This outfit requires dry-cleaning. I'm asking to be sprayed with blood or vomit, aren't I?"

"I'd say that's about right. If you get bled on, you'll have no one but yourself to blame."

I felt better after lunch. That is, until I was accosted by Barb. She dragged me into an empty examination room and closed the door. I turned to face her worried gaze.

"Pam, a good friend of mine, Stan Lieberman, is scheduled to see you for groin pain. It started after that strong wind we had a couple of days ago. He was trying to keep a fence from falling down. Dr. Bachelder saw him about a year and a half ago for epididymitis and his wife says he's had persistent swelling in that left testicle since then. He refused to be re-checked, figuring it was normal to be a little large all this time, especially

182

since he's had absolutely no pain, and he was a hurting puppy with that epididymitis."

Alarms went off in my head. "Normal for a year and a half?" I asked incredulously. "Is his wife here?"

"No. He didn't want her to come, but she was afraid he might not mention it, so she called and asked that I talk to you."

"Based on what you're telling me, I don't think I'll miss the problem."

"So, Mr. Lieberman," I remarked nonchalantly, closing the door behind me a few moments later, "I understand you fought the wind to save a fence the other day and you've been having pain since. Is that right?"

"Yes. I wouldn't have come in today except it's really bothering me."

As I put on my gloves, I casually asked, "Do you check your testicles every month for suspicious lumps?"

"No. I'm only thirty-four, and other than my left one still being a bit enlarged from the epididymitis I had about eighteen months ago, I haven't noticed any problems."

I turned to face him. "Testicular cancer is a problem that can turn up before you're thirty-four. One of our patients was only fifteen when he was diagnosed. Men should check their testicles every month, just like women check their breasts. If you feel uncomfortable doing it yourself, you can ask your wife to check you."

"I think I can manage," he grinned, lowering his trousers and underwear.

Stan's testicle was the size of a billiard ball, round, and very firm. A small bulge was evident in his left groin.

"I think we are, indeed, looking at a small hernia," I said after finishing his exam. "But to be honest, that isn't what concerns me right now. This left testicle is not normal, and I know it could not have been this large and firm when Dr. Bachelder saw you a year and a half ago."

"Well, it may be a little larger."

I looked at the note Gloria had written in his chart. "Patient was instructed to return for re-check if symptoms have not completely abated in two weeks." Denial can be a powerful force.

"I'm going to phone a urologist, Mr. Lieberman. I want an appointment for you within twenty-four hours."

"What do you think is going on?"

"I'm not going to lie to you. A non-tender mass like that is not good. I need to rule out cancer."

His face fell. "It could be cancer?"

"I hope I'm wrong, sir, but cancer's a strong possibility at this point. The diagnosis needs to be confirmed. I'll schedule an ultrasound this afternoon, and you and your wife need to see a urologist tomorrow."

"Cancer?" he said again quietly. Several seconds later he asked, "Will you call my wife? She's been nagging me for months to get checked, but I was too stubborn."

I walked out to the nurse's station to ask Barb to schedule a stat ultrasound. I called Mr. Lieberman's wife. She'd suspected for months, but she'd been unable to drag him to the office.

"I couldn't very well bring his testicle without him, could I?" she asked. "Although I was tempted to do just that many times, believe me. Tell Stan I'll be there in about twenty minutes. Will we be able to talk to you before we leave the office?"

"Of course. When you arrive, ask the front desk to page me. I'll come talk to you and your husband as quickly as possible."

"Thank-you," she whispered. "Is Barb there? Would it be possible to speak to her?"

After Barb replaced the receiver, she turned to me. "Cancer?"

"I hope to God I'm wrong, Barb. But I don't think so, and we have to assume the worst to ensure he gets in to the specialist quickly. Most men don't check their testicles every month like they should."

I let Stan know his wife would be arriving shortly. For what must have been the hundredth time, I heard a patient tell me that s/he figured it "couldn't be serious, because it didn't hurt". I wished there were some way to tell people that if they had a firm lump that didn't go away within a couple of weeks, it should be checked whether it hurt or not. Most of the time, lumps proved to be benign fibro- adenomas, lipomas, sebaceous cysts, or the like, but unless a patient was confident about the diagnosis, it was better to check with a health care provider.

Taking a deep breath, I pulled the next patient's chart out of the rack beside the door and entered the room. He was new to the clinic, I noted. Gray-haired and smiling, Mr. Benson wore a Bronco's T-shirt. He extended his hand in greeting.

I introduced myself. "Hello, Mr. Benson. Broncos' fan, huh?"

"Yeah, I love the Broncos. I even painted my old VW bus orange and blue. I did it just before they won the first Super Bowl game two years ago.

I have a few Broncos' flags hanging out the windows. I'm a big fan. I also work for the team."

"That's terrific. It's important to support the local team, whether they play poorly or win the Super Bowl. Although I'm not a great football fan, my husband loves the game, so I concentrate on the parts of the game that interest me. Some of the players have great tight ends, if you know what I mean, and I'm not talking about a football position. My husband enjoys his action and I enjoy mine. You say you work for the Broncos? Cool! What do you do?"

"Well, I'm a pastor in Denver; I have my own parish, but I also occasionally minister to the team. Once in a while, I go on the road with them, although there is another fellow that works with the Broncos full-time."

"A minister, huh? I guess I didn't score any points talking about those tight ends. Sorry." My face flamed.

Mr. Benson laughed. "That's okay. I take life pretty light-heartedly. You didn't offend me at all."

"How can I help you today?" I tried to recover my professionalism.

"My throat is really sore. I can hardly swallow. I've been running a fever and feel miserable. And there's white stuff on my tonsils. Oh, by the way, could you check something else for me? Since you were talking about tight ends and all. I've experienced occasional rectal bleeding the last few months. Sometimes there's just a bit of blood on the tissue."

"Do you have hemorrhoids?"

"I don't think so. But it's been painful to sit down for weeks."

"Is there a family history of colon cancer?"

"My father and one of his brothers had colon cancer."

"How old were they when diagnosed with colon cancer?"

"Dad was sixty-three at the time. I'm not sure how old my uncle was."

"And you are fifty-eight now. Have you been scoped to check for colon polyps?"

He shook his head.

"I'll check you for hemorrhoids today, but with your family history, it's imperative that you have a colonoscopy to rule out polyps. Colon polyps precede colon cancer. Bright red blood may indicate hemorrhoids, but even if my exam confirms you have some, I'd like you to proceed with the colon test. I'll write a referral."

"I heard about those scopes, doctor. Isn't that where they put a tube up your, uh…." he stammered.

"Yes, they do. They can examine the tissue with a camera that's attached to the physician's end of the scope. It's really important you have this done. In fact, we generally recommend the first colon exam at age fifty, especially with a family history like yours. Please follow through with the colonoscopy. It's not the most pleasant test to think about, but you'll be given sedation to help you through it."

"Okay, okay, doctor," Mr. Benson laughed, throwing up his hands. "You've convinced me. I'll get scoped."

"Good. Just in case you missed it when I introduced myself, though, I am a nurse practitioner, not a doctor."

"I didn't miss it. But you see the same patients the doctors do, right?"

"That's right. Let me review your past medical history and the rest of your family history, and then I'll attend to your sore throat and your sore other end."

"Okay and thanks."

After his exam, I headed into the nurse's station and picked up a bottle of hemoccult developer from the drawer. I opened the card on which I had deposited a small stool sample and placed a drop of solution on each side. I held the card up to a light to check for hidden blood. Barb, knowing I had gone into the room to see a patient with a sore throat, asked, "Where did you go for that throat culture?"

"Cute, Barb! This was an 'oh by the way.' How often do we get asked about other problems when we see a patient?"

"How often do we *not* get asked about other problems would be the more logical question," Dr. Bachelder chuckled, walking into the nurses' station. "How are you feeling today, Pam?"

"Tired, but otherwise okay. Thanks for asking. I am bummed that my hair is thinning by the day. Jon uncharitably remarked that everyone knows where I've been, because my hair is all over the house. The sad news is he's right. It's depressing. I wouldn't mind so much if it would grow back in a lovely auburn or blond shade, but I think it'll remain gray. Dr. Sitarik said hair texture might change after chemo. With my luck, I told him, it would probably look like pubic hair. He said that happens sometimes. I was joking, but he didn't even crack a smile. Imagine the jokes if my head looks like a pubis. I'll be a little old lady with gray pubic hair on my head. What I wouldn't give to go back a few years."

"You aren't the only one who would like to turn back the hands of time, Pam," Dr. Bachelder countered. "I'm going to be thirty-eight this year."

"Ooh! We've got ourselves a positively ancient broad here."

"I know I'm not the oldest one around," Gloria Bachelder retorted, "but I would like to get pregnant before my thirty-ninth birthday."

"Hey, don't tell me! That is information you should share with your husband. You think you're old? My baby is going to be eighteen tomorrow." I could hardly believe it.

"But at least you've had three kids," Gloria chided. "I'm not greedy; I'd just like one more."

A horrendous noise originated from Room 1. "What is that obscene sound?" I asked.

"The autoclave is acting up," Gail remarked. "Like everything else around here, it's falling apart. I just came from the kitchen. Did you know there's a trapdoor in the kitchen floor to allow access to pipes? No one bothered to tell the nurses that a plumber would be working on the pipes today. I almost fell in the hole. Speaking of kitchen, does anyone know where we can get a cheap second-hand refrigerator? Ours has died and can not be resurrected, according to the repairman."

"Is there anything that still works around here?" I interjected.

"Certainly not the providers by the looks of things," responded Gail. A smile tugged at the corners of her mouth as she scanned the faces of two doctors and me clustered in the nurse's station.

"The abuse we take around here is unbelievable," Dr. Hibbard challenged.

"And well deserved, doctor," Gail added, laughing.

"Well, as far as I can tell, if we didn't have such great providers no one would come to this dilapidated clinic," I responded, semi-seriously.

"Let's see if you can break your arm patting yourself on the back," Gail teased. "What do we nurses look like, chopped liver? Where do you think all of you would be if we didn't keep things running smoothly for you?"

"I'm glad we have such a mutual admiration society," I joked. Gail was right, as usual.

"Pam, Room 2," a voice rang out on the paging system in the nurse's station.

"I'm right here," I said looking directly at Barb, the pager.

"Yeah, but I don't want you right here," Barb quipped. "I want you to see the patient in Room 2."

"On my way, master." I saluted. I don't know how I would have made it through each day without Barb's good-natured razzing. "Just let me tell Mr. Benson the news that his hemoccult is positive for blood and give him some instructions about caring for both ends of his GI system until he gets scoped."

I had completed my third Pap in a row when Sophia, from the front desk, popped her head into the nurse's station.

"Pam, we have a walk-in: a ten-year-old kid with a laceration. You only have a fifteen-minute opening, but do you think you could squeeze him in? Or should we send him to the urgent care up the street?"

"Put him in Room 1. I'm taking a lot of flack about not being busy enough today, jawing with the docs. See if you can keep me busy the rest of the afternoon. Maybe I can redeem myself in the nurses' eyes, but I doubt it."

I turned to Barb. "I knew there was no way I could avoid blood or vomit on this new outfit. That'll teach me to wear nice clothes around here."

I meandered to Room 1, and while the boy's mother filled out the consent form, I casually asked my patient, Phillip, how he cut himself.

His grin stretched from ear to ear. "I was bitten by a shark in my aunt's car."

I laughed. "Okay, I'll bite—no pun intended. How did a shark bite you in your aunt's car?"

"My cousin, Jimmy, borrowed this shark's jaw from his dad who caught a Reef shark off the coast of Florida a few years ago. Jimmy wanted to show the shark's teeth to his class. When I got into the car, I slipped and fell on the shark's jaw. I cut my knee. It really hurts."

"I'll bet it does. I'll fix you up in a jiffy. Would you mind if I share your little story with the nurses after we sew you up?" I rummaged through cabinets to extract supplies.

"Sure; go ahead and tell 'em."

After cleaning the wound, I began suturing. The boy's mother turned a ghastly shade of pale.

"Mrs. Rogers, please sit down now," I commanded.

"I'm okay," Mrs. Rogers replied, whitening to the color of an anemic ghost. "My son needs me to hold his hand."

"Ma'am, your son is fine." I became alarmed. "Please sit down now. You can hold your son's hand while you're seated." The woman started to wobble. I jumped up, ripped off my gloves and reached Phillip's mother as she fainted.

In response to my call, Barb and Gail ran in.

"Is my mom going to be okay?" Phillip asked alarmed, as the two nurses helped the woman to another room to lie down.

"She'll be fine, just like you will be. A lot of parents have trouble watching their kids get sewn up. I've gotten dizzy myself when my children's cuts were being repaired."

"No kidding! Wow! Did you ever pass out?"

"No, but I came pretty close. It's hard to watch someone you love get stitches."

I checked Phillip's mother's blood pressure, returned to Room 1, put on a new pair of gloves, and kept up a running inventory of clean jokes—not easy, believe me—while I finished sewing up Phillip's knee. He was a trooper.

"I'll put a bandage on your knee and check on your mom once more. When she's feeling better, I'll tell her how to care for your shark bite and watch for infection. Then you guys can go home. You came through this better than she did."

"Yeah, I did great!"

A short person accosted me in the hallway. He wrapped his arms tightly around my legs. "Pam!"

"Good afternoon, Anthony." I tousled the four-year-old's thick black hair. "You're wearing new sneakers."

"Look, Pam. The light turns on when I walk." He walked away from me, each step accompanied by an eerie red glow on the heel of his shoes.

"That's really cool. Do you think your shoes would fit me?"

"No, silly!" Anthony roared. "We're going to get a puppy today!"

"What kind?"

"A black one."

I told everyone Anthony was my boyfriend. I'd been seeing him for well-child checks and sick visits since he was two. All my boyfriends were under the age of five—so far. I told Bill I preferred younger men, but I rarely got more than a sneer from him. He knew me too well.

"Anthony was hoping you'd be in today, Pam," his mother explained. "He wanted to show you his new shoes before we pick up our Labrador retriever."

"I'm always happy to see my favorite boyfriend." I gave him a hug and a sticker from the box at the front desk and waved at him as he left.

"You're fickle, Pam," Gloria Bachelder snickered. "I know for a fact you have more than one favorite boyfriend in this clinic, including my son, Nicholas."

She was right, of course.

After checking Phillip's mom—now a healthier color—I saw Mr. Adams, an elderly gentleman with a significant hearing loss. He regularly saw Dr. Richard for care of his diabetes. Since Tuesday was Dr. Richard's day off, Mr. Adams was mine for the day. Dr. Richard had unsuccessfully urged Mr. Adams to buy a hearing aid for years. A putrid odor assailed my nostrils as I entered the room.

"What can I do for you, Mr. Adams?" I asked in a loud voice, hoping I wouldn't have to raise my voice too much.

"Huh?" Mr. Adams responded.

Sure the entire clinic would hear our conversation, I repeated louder, "What can I do for you, Mr. Adams?"

"Huh?"

I need a megaphone, I thought, shouting the question into his ear.

Silently he removed his sock and pointed to the warm, red area on the top of his foot. Just as silently, I put on a glove and picked up his foot. I noticed a moist area on the floor where it had been resting. Gently, I turned his foot so I could look at the bottom. I'd found the source of the putrid smell. An area of necrosis—dead tissue—surrounded a hole on the bottom of his foot.

My stomach lurched. "Mr. Adams, do you ever look at the bottoms of your feet?"

"Huh?"

"Do you ever look at the bottoms of your feet?" I shouted into his ear.

"Not too often. Dr. Richard is forever telling me to check my feet, because diabetics lose feeling in them, but I don't think about it much. Is something wrong?"

I showed him the wound. "We need to admit you to the hospital," I hollered.

"Huh?"

"We need to admit you to the hospital," I screeched into his ear.

"Is that really necessary? I don't much like hospitals."

"It's necessary," I shouted. "We would like you to keep your foot if possible. If this doesn't heal, it will need to be amputated."

"Lord, have mercy, do whatever you have to!"

I called for a medical bed at Boulder Community Hospital before searching for Dr. Pittenger, who was on-call, to discuss orders. Sharon Pittenger was one of my favorite docs—okay, they were all sort of my favorites, just like the masses of cute, curly-headed males under the age of five. Sharon was easy-going, kind, and a great listener. She was also Irish, so we shared information about area Irish events. After we finalized orders for Mr. Adams, I passed the front desk on the way to my office. A beautiful arrangement of flowers graced the counter.

"Those are beautiful," I gushed. "Who are they for?"

Tricia glanced up from her computer and looked at the card. "As hard as it is to believe, they're for you, Pam."

"Cool!"

I opened the card as Tricia hovered nearby. "A secret admirer or not so secret lover, perhaps, Pam?"

"Oh, sure, and when am I supposed to have time to see someone on the side? I have trouble keeping up with the one I have at home. No, they're from a patient, if you want to know." I fingered the card. "You know, Tricia, maybe I will tell Bill these are from an admirer. It might make the evening more interesting."

"Bill will never buy it, Pam. I heard about your confrontation with the drug rep at lunchtime. Who's going to be interested in a middle-aged nurse practitioner with attitude?"

"Ooh, bite me!"

"All kidding aside, except for your tiredness, you seem to be holding up pretty well. How many treatments have you had?"

"Four and counting down. And at least I still have some of my hair." A look of horror crossed Tricia's face. "What did I say?" I demanded. Tricia pointed behind me. I turned quickly, nearly tripping over Regina Sheridan. Mrs. Sheridan, a seventy-five year old patient of Dr. Hibbard's, had chronic alopecia and had been bald for over twenty years.

"Gosh, Mrs. Sheridan, I didn't know you were behind me," I stammered. "I wasn't comparing my hair loss to yours. Oh, good grief." I steered the surprised woman to an exam room, figuring I wouldn't be able to extricate my foot from my mouth without explaining about my own hair loss from chemo. As I closed the door, I could make out the poorly stifled guffaws of the women at the front desk.

Barb was strangling with laughter as I walked back to the nurse's station. "You have a patient in Room 2," she gasped.

"May I assume," I mentioned casually, "that you and the rest of the clinic have already heard about what happened with Mrs. Sheridan?"

"You may, Pam," Barb managed to get out between bouts of choked sniggering.

"Fine. And just for the record, I didn't know she was standing behind me when I made the comment about losing hair."

"Sure, Pam. That's almost as good as that ridiculous comment you made to the patient with the auburn hair."

"Oh, God. I'd forgotten about that."

"Ha! That's one of those momentous occasions you will never forget."

"You're right. I still think about it, and the poor patient probably remembers it now and again as well."

There weren't many patient situations I re-ran through my brain on a regular basis, but there've been a few times I accidentally embarrassed a patient, and I had trouble forgiving myself. Believe me, I tried to keep patients comfortable during clinic visits. Paps were tough appointments for many women. I kept up a running commentary while I examined them, trying to prevent their fixating on the reason for their visits. During one exam, I commented on a patient's beautiful auburn hair. She made no remark during the rest of the Pap. It wasn't until she sat up that I remembered the hair on her head had been dyed black.

Gil Peters lay on the exam table in room 2, groaning and holding his stomach.

"Hi, Mr. Peters. What's going on?"

"Oh, I'm hurting so bad."

"When did your pain start?"

"Last night after dinner."

"What did you have for dinner, Mr. Peters?"

"A few tacos with hot picante sauce, some refried beans, and a few beers."

"How many beers are we talking about?"

"No more than six or eight. We were watching the ballgame—me and some buddies. You know how that goes. Ohh, God, am I hurting!"

"According to your chart, you have a history of PUD."

"What's that?" Gil gasped.

"Peptic ulcer disease. It says here you had a stomach ulcer and were treated for H. pylori bacterial infection, which accounts for many of the ulcers we see."

"Yeah, that's right, but that was last year and I've been doing pretty well. Make it stop hurting, please! I really have trouble when I eat Mexican food or drink booze."

"I hate stating the obvious, but stop eating Mexican food and drinking booze."

"Get serious, please! They're my favorites. Can't you give me a pill to pop so I can eat whatever I want? I tried a Pepcid AC last night but it didn't help much."

"You are way beyond Pepcid AC, Mr. Peters. Have you been spitting up blood?"

"Not really. Well maybe once. Just a little, but not like the time I had the ulcer."

"I'll check you and put you on medication to decrease stomach acid production, but you have to seriously consider permanent diet changes. If you aren't feeling better in the next few days, or if there is further bleeding, please call the clinic or on-call doctor immediately. Okay?"

We talked about diet changes before I examined him. Near the end of the exam, I said, "Please put this drape over your lap, pull your trousers down, and roll on your left side so I can do a rectal exam."

"Is that necessary?"

"It is. If it isn't your favorite part of a medical exam, remember it the next time you're eating tacos and beer." I snapped on a pair of gloves.

Tricia called my name as I passed the front desk.

"Pam, I have a lady on line 2. She was cleaning her ear with a Q-tip when her daughter opened the bathroom door and smashed her elbow. The Q-tip was shoved into her ear. When she pulled it out, her ear bled. Should I have her go to the urgent care or come here? I realize it's time to go home."

I sighed. I was exhausted, and that was the only reason I could come up with later for uttering my inappropriate remark. "No, I'll see her. Tell her to get her butt over here as soon as possible, okay?"

Tricia spoke into the phone. "Ma'am, Pam says if you get your butt over here right away, she'll see you." Tricia glanced up at a family nurse practitioner whose gut had suddenly twisted in a knot. I'm sure my face mirrored my inner horror that such a thoughtless comment would be conveyed to a patient.

"Got you," laughed Tricia. "I wish I had a camera. Actually, the patient is still on hold. I just wanted to see how you would respond if you thought I conveyed your 'butt' comment."

I began breathing again. "What is this? Pick on Pam day?" I laughed.

"Aw, you're just such an easy target, Pam. We have to take you down a peg or two once in a while."

"My peg has already been taken down a couple of notches today, thank-you very much. Let me know when the patient arrives. I'll be in my office finishing charts and eating crow."

Chapter 23 - April 4th

The whole family attended Mass on Easter. I almost didn't recognize the men in my life when they trotted down the stairs. They wore suits, were freshly shaven and smelled of cologne—actually, Rob smelled like he'd bathed in the stuff. Heather had bought me a corsage. The day was gloriously clear and my heart felt light and thankful.

We got to the church early to beat out all the C&E Catholics—members of the faithful who attended Mass only at Christmas and Easter. I'll admit I occasionally drifted toward joining their ranks. Our small church accommodated regular churchgoers, but it was standing room only on those two holy days. However, I imagined our priest didn't mind a few extra bucks in the collection plate.

After praying, I pondered the promise inherent in resurrection. I experienced a surge of hope, grateful for my life, and all it still might be—whether or not future accomplishments would be in this life or the next. Dozens of fragrant Easter lilies surrounding the altar symbolized a belief that God would continue to be at my side.

In the pew before me, a mother cuddled a five- or six-month-old baby to her shoulder. His bright eyes returned many times to my face. I smiled and furtively waved. I was rewarded with toothless grins and tiny gurgles.

"Cut that out!" Bill begged. "You'll give Heather ideas."

"Isn't he cute? I need one of those."

"Oh, no, you don't! We have three dogs already. I forbid you to get into your 'I want another baby mood' that will end up in our buying another dog."

"Relax. There's a three-dog limit in Louisville. But he is cute, isn't he?"

"He's darling, just as long as he goes home with someone else."

"Shh!" Heather scolded, semi-seriously. "You're always telling *us* not to talk in church."

I sat repentant until I could sneak in additional waves at the baby boy. I tried to concentrate during Mass, but my mind drifted to patients I'd seen the week before. I'd be off this next week, the middle week of my treatment cycle, and I knew I'd worry about a few patients. To ease my guilt-ridden mind, I haunted the clinic two or three evenings during the weeks I was off to review labs and call patients.

The cantor began singing *Jesus Is Risen* and jolted my mind back to Mass. Jon and Rob stifled laughs with difficulty. Soon Bill and Heather joined in. Even I couldn't help snickering. That hymn would do us all in, and it was Rowan Atkinson's fault.

In *Rowan Atkinson Live!* on HBO, the comedian set a slightly irreverent skit in church. A rendition of *Jesus Is Risen* complemented the performance. The comedian nearly fell asleep during the service while the minister droned on. Rowan kept his bulging eyes open by prying them apart with his fingers, and then he spent several minutes noisily unwrapping a piece of candy, which he tried, unsuccessfully, to maneuver to his mouth.

My family collapsed with laughter every time we watched the tape. And, of course, hearing that hymn brought the skit to mind. We stifled our giggling with unbelievable difficulty—as did the couple directly in front of us. When it came time to greet others in the congregation, the couple turned to us and asked, "Rowan Atkinson fans?" We lost it once more.

Surely we'd be confessing our irreverent behavior during the next week or two. "Bless me father, for I have sinned. My last confession was a week ago. I laughed during Mass. And if you don't stop selecting *Jesus Is Risen* to be sung for the rest of the Easter season, I'll be in here again next week."

When we left church, Rob declared, "If Mass could be fun like that all the time, I'd go more often."

"You don't go to Mass to enjoy yourself," Bill half-joked. "Did you see that dirty look your mother gave us? I noticed she did a poor job keeping a straight face, however."

"A little decorum at Mass would have been appropriate," I said. "But I admit it was funny. They always sing that same hymn for weeks after Easter. We'll all be in trouble for the next few Sundays."

We explored the church cemetery before getting into the car and driving into Boulder for breakfast.

I'd planned a rib roast for dinner, so I had plenty of time to read, reflect, and nap. As soon as we arrived home, the kids scattered, each having made arrangements to spend the afternoon with friends so Mom could have some "quiet time". They promised help with dinner, but I'd believe that when I saw it. Bill holed up in his office for the afternoon revising protocols for work. Gross!

I propped myself up in bed. That way, if exhaustion overcame me, I could just scoot down and pass out. Before torturing myself with my daily language lesson—I was trying to learn some Irish verb conjugations—I thought about phone calls I'd received from patients who had weathered their own bouts of cancer. They'd bolstered my sagging spirits and volunteered to accompany me to any of the many cancer support groups available in the Boulder-Denver area. Their kindness moved me to tears, emotionally labile that I still was, but I was not yet ready to accept their generosity. The comradery on the phone was grand, as were the lunches shared, but I was far from ready to join a support group. Support groups helped many men and women face their trials with grace and sanity. I faced those trials with my patients—holding them, listening to them, and crying with them—but I felt emotionally unable to bear more grief than that. Away from work, I surrounded myself with as many light diversions as possible.

I felt bombarded at work. I'd been evaluating more patients with breast lumps. "My friend recommended that I see you. She thought you'd understand what I'm going through," they'd say. I understood, but they had no idea how my gut churned and bile rose in my throat thinking this might be a woman who would face the same diagnosis. Please, God, I'd beg, make this one benign. Please! It took enormous effort to call a woman whose tests were suspicious and choke out the words that stuck in my throat. It required all my reserve to hold back my own flood of tears when I held her in an exam room, encouraging verbalization of her consuming panic after hearing the dreaded diagnosis of cancer.

I got them into the hospitals for their ultrasounds and mammograms quickly. I knew that a week or two would make no difference in the overall prognosis, but mentally, a week or two was an eternity when facing a cloudy future. The docs I worked with were every bit as speedy as I was in getting patients scheduled for tests, but patients verbalized their beliefs that I knew how they felt, since I was "going through it". Unfortunately I did. I had always cared—always, as did the docs at Family Medical Center.

I experienced emotional pulls toward ladies who knew, as I had, that their lives would irrevocably change with a diagnosis of breast cancer. At the same time, I wanted to pull away from them. Their suffering—both physical and emotional—took a poignant toll on me, and although I'd read a few magazine stories about women who claimed cancer did not change them, I realized my life was changed forever.

Changes evolved slowly, but they became increasingly evident to a woman who had a Type A personality. Like so many working mothers, I obligated myself to more activities than I could comfortably handle. "No" was not part of my vocabulary, but I occasionally experienced short bursts of temper when I couldn't handle the stress—like it was everybody else's fault I obligated myself to the brink of despair. Most people thought me nice enough—although there have definitely been a few personalities that clashed with mine.

I rarely took the time to appreciate the world around me or give thanks to God for leading me into nursing. I truly believe He had a hand in it. After graduating from high school, I planned a career in advertising—a career that would have easily afforded greater financial rewards. But I'd taken a course in advertising the summer before I started college, and I knew it was not what I was meant to do. I'd spent the rest of the summer questioning and praying about my choice. One day, about six weeks into the fall semester of college, I was in a shoe store and spotted a pair of nursing shoes. I burst into tears. I realized that was where I'd been headed my whole life.

I'd resisted the idea of becoming a nurse. My mother was a nurse, and she shared the difficulties inherent in the profession. It was emotionally and physically draining, she'd told my sister and me. Often the respect that was well deserved had come from within, because many physicians and patients considered nurses intellectually inferior—some still did, which was one of the reasons I felt so blessed working with the doctors I did.

I treasured the memory of the call to my mother when I told her I was changing my college major to nursing. She'd shown up unannounced four hours later (it took three hours and forty-five minutes to get to my dorm from our home in Fayetteville, North Carolina), and she'd spent a couple of days talking to me to make sure I knew "what I was getting into". During my college years, I never regretted my decision and had only occasionally questioned my sanity since then, usually when I was so tired I could barely stand. And it all began over a pair of nursing shoes—perhaps I should say the idea was cemented then, because the thought germinated in my subconscious long before.

As demanding as my profession had always been (and few nurses would disagree that nursing exacted great emotional and physical tolls), I felt honored giving comfort to people needing compassion and guidance. But instead of appreciating that I had so many opportunities to help others, I found myself, in recent years, collapsing at the end of each workday, questioning why I put myself through the rigors of surrounding myself with people who were sick, grumpy, angry, frightened, or depressed. No one ever made an appointment because he or she was having a terrific day and just wanted to bring sunshine into my life. Feeling overwhelmed by a particularly baffling case or an emotionally gut-wrenching patient visit left me worried and cranky. That was *never* the way I wished to present myself to patients, but it happened now and again. Nurses are human too.

However, I'd been the happy recipient of many bouquets of flowers, baskets of fruits and goodies, letters of appreciation, and free lunches through the years. Nursing pay was pitiful, but the perks were emotionally rewarding. Prayers were always appreciated. One of my patients from Virginia Beach still sent cards at Christmas, letting me know I was remembered in some novena or another. Her thoughtfulness touched me. She had come to see me for an annual Pap, and I found a lesion that proved to be cancerous. She was grateful, and I'd been the lucky recipient of her prayers for years. God obviously missed her prayer the day my first breast cancer cell split in two, but He's a busy guy.

Cancer slowed down my hectic life. I relaxed more and worried less. I had little reserve energy to agonize over much outside my health. I no longer wished time would fly when I experienced overwhelming physical or psychological distress. I appreciated each patient, each friend, each hour of my day—most of the time. I decreased my commitments to enjoy the few I had energy to complete. I didn't feel as guilty when I had to say, "No".

Perspectives changed. I no longer thought about being old at fifty. If I made it to fifty, it would be over four years since my diagnosis. That day would find me celebrating in Galway, Ireland, since a dear friend offered her home whenever I felt the pull toward her native country.

Speaking of Ireland, it was time to stop daydreaming and study. I'd told Bill to wake me if I failed to materialize downstairs by two o'clock. Before then, I wanted to study Irish. When I'd begun studying the language, I'd naively thought it would be easy, since I'd sailed through four years of French in high school. Ha!

I should have known there'd be trouble when I decided to learn the parts of the body. Dutifully echoing the pronunciation of my on-line Irish teacher—Jon bought a computer program for my birthday—I looked at the word for face (*aghaidh*) and heard the teacher pronounce those seven letters as a long "i". That was it—"i"!

I figured out what happened, of course. Long ago, Irish and Welsh forefathers shared a few pints and decided how to split up their respective branches of the ancient Celtic language.

"Our mutual goal should be to combine letters into as many diphthongs and triphthongs as possible, so nobody knows what the hell we're saying. You Irish use as many vowels as possible, and we'll use more consonants. Determining rules of conjugation should take a few days. After you've come up with the rules, let them set in your mind for a few weeks, have a few more pints, and then agree on as many exceptions to the rules as is humanly possible. That way, when some poor *eejit* tries to write a grammatical text centuries from now, he'll receive a tidy bit of compensation for making sense of the whole thing." I made that up, but it surely could have happened.

Having said all that, I have to backtrack and say I've been unfair. Not unfair in the language department, because Irish is tough, and learning it has given me an entirely new appreciation for the intelligence of the race, but in the "few extra pints" department. The Irish have been saddled with a raw deal concerning alcohol. Various sources have placed the Irish per capita consumption as somewhere between third and seventh in Western Europe. They're at least behind the English and my German ancestors. In fact, there are many Irish teetotalers. The Irish Capuchin monk from County Cork who promoted temperance, Father Theobald Mathew, is remembered with a statue on O'Connell Street in Dublin. He's earned his bit of immortality, since his name and likeness are splashed across town squares, town halls, and streets around the Republic.

The Irish have many delightful sayings deploring the drink. My favorite is: "Drink is the curse of the land. It makes you fight with your neighbor, shoot at your landlord, and makes you miss your target." In Ireland, a pub is a social environment where friends meet, share news and gossip, and avoid confrontations, *nappies* (diapers), and late night infant feedings at home.

I'm not sure whether or not a couple of pints would help my grasp of the language, but I was determined to learn Irish. I figured I'd know enough in ten years to get into trouble. How hard could it be? Even a word borrowed from English, like *bus*, takes on a life and pronunciation of its own depending on the words preceding it. One may say "on the bus" (*ar on mbus*—pronounced moos) but "in the bus" (*sa bhus*—pronounced woos). Go figure.

And no, most of the words didn't look anything like English. Heather came home one afternoon and asked to borrow one of my Irish dictionaries. She couldn't convince her pals that the Irish people had a language of their own. "How hard it is to speak Irish?" they demanded. "All you've got to do is speak English with an Irish accent." Lord, give me strength.

My friends didn't understand my fascination with the language, but I'd always been interested in ancient forms of communication like Latin, Aramaic, and Egyptian. Irish was an ancient language that was banned for centuries by the English. The language survived because areas of the western province, Connaught, were too isolated and poor to merit invasion or pillaging. Sheep grazing and turf cutting sustained the small population living in the rocky, bog-covered province. The English damned their enemies to "hell or Connaught". It was left to those living in remote regions to preserve and cherish the native customs and tongue.

Once southern Ireland gained independence, the old ways were embraced. Those living in the *Gaeltacht* (parts of Connaught and other small provincial pockets of human isolation that spoke the language) were sought out by learned scholars. Now, every school kid in the Republic spends years learning Irish, but few adults speak it regularly. It's a beautiful language—subtle, mystical, poetic, and warm.

Thinking about the history of the language would not help me learn it, so I stuck in a *Buntús Cainte, part 1* tape into my cassette recorder and vowed to spend serious time studying. I probably confused myself studying one Irish program on-line and a totally different program when I rested in bed, but I hoped one or the other teaching styles would one day make sense.

Sometime during my Herculean effort to master another bit of Irish, I dozed off. Bill's voice penetrated my dream. "Honey, you told me to wake you up when it was time to put the roast in the oven."

"Go raibh maith agat, Liam. Tiocfaidh mé díreach anois, ach ba mhaith liom dul a chodladh tar éis dinnéar, le do thoil." ("Thank-you, Bill. I will come right away, but I would like to sleep after dinner, please.") Okay, it didn't come out quite that clear. It probably wasn't even close, but it's what I *would* have said. Bill looked at me like I had rocks in my head, but he helped me with dinner, and the children cleaned up the dishes so I could go back to sleep.

Chapter 24 - April 16th

Treatment number five aroused mixed feelings. Treatments were nearly over, and I should have been elated, yet depression consumed me. I couldn't pinpoint the origin of my sadness. Perhaps my subconscious realized there would be at least six more weeks of side effects before facing the unknown of radiation—and there were bound to be physical reactions associated with that therapy as well. The whole process was getting old.

Until chemotherapy and radiation treatments were completed, I knew cancer would permeate my daily thoughts, no matter how much I tried to avoid thinking about it. When patients and friends asked how I felt, it took all my effort to smile and say, "I'm fine—no worries." Co-workers commented on my cheerful attitude and sometimes marveled at my inner strength. Right. My inner strength was a façade. I was still very scared.

I relished each hour that I didn't feel like I'd walked a hundred miles and been drop kicked over a cliff for good measure. To be honest, there weren't many good hours these days. After the next treatment, I'd feel even worse. Pushing the thought from my consciousness, I thought of Bill, our future, and our kids as I stared at the traffic outside the window of the exam room waiting for Dr. Sitarik.

I turned from the window as he walked into the room.

"Your blood counts look okay, Pam. The white count's a bit lower than on previous visits, but overall, acceptable. You should do fine with your treatment—physically, that is. You look sad today, though."

"I feel sorry for myself again today. You must tire of dealing with depressed people, Dr. Sitarik."

"It's hard sometimes, but it goes with the job. Are you experiencing increasing side effects?"

"Fatigue is wiping me out. My whole body, especially my mucous membranes, feels dry. I use saline eye drops several times a day. Mouth ulcers plague me, but I neglected to take my folic acid at least half of the past three weeks. My hair is thinning like crazy. I'm experiencing hot and cold flashes, so I spend my day putting on sweaters and ripping them off. The girls at work think I'm possessed. What else can I complain about? Ah, yes. My boobs feel lumpier than usual. Can that be a side effect of these treatments?"

He smiled. "Yes, lumpy breasts can be a problem. I'll check them today. Anything else?"

"The skin of my neck, face, and chest has reddened more. And as the *pièce de résistance*, I spend half my day in the bathroom with diarrhea. That's all. Compared to women taking more toxic drugs, I have nothing to complain about. Yet here I am grumbling. I don't know what's wrong with me today. Maybe it's the weather. It looks like it may snow again, even though it was 65 degrees less than thirty-six hours ago."

"It's Colorado," he commented. "You know what they say—if you don't like the weather, wait five minutes."

"I've heard that."

"Any other concerns today?"

"I could use some suggestions for winning numbers in the state lotto."

"Sorry. My track record in that department leaves something to be desired."

"Fine. I guess I'm ready for my treatment."

"Good." He stepped outside while I changed. Returning a few minutes later, he said, "Hop up on the exam table. I have no scientific data to back up this observation, but I've noticed many patients reach their emotional nadir just before the fifth treatment. I'm not sure why."

I pondered his comment as he examined me. The side effects, especially the fatigue, had significantly increased the past couple of weeks. Bill had taken over more of my home duties and pressed the kids into service, but it was still all I could do to drag myself out of bed each morning. Bill's willingness to continue helping around the house was an unexpected bonus in my fight, and I liked it very much.

I begged off the Decadron for this treatment. The steroid gave me three to four sleepless nights, despite a trial of sleeping pills that just drugged me the next day. It didn't completely prevent nausea and made me ravenous. I had to fight a desire to clean out the refrigerator every time I ate. I'd gained four pounds in the past three weeks because I was too tired to exercise most days—despite my earlier assertion that I'd crawl on the treadmill rather than gain weight. I felt like a big fat slob with cancer.

I wondered if I could make myself any more depressed as I walked down the hall to the treatment room. I forced one foot in front of the other and thought about my depleted white blood cell count. Since it was now below normal, I was more susceptible to illness, and this was *before* my treatment. God only knew what it would be like in ten days. Irresponsibly,

I neglected to mention the chills I'd experienced for two days. I had no other symptoms, but chills might be heralding an illness. Of course, chills might be another side effect. I should have told Dr. Sitarik, but I was afraid he might put off today's treatment, and I was desperate to finish—two more treatments including today, then radiation and after that, the promise of getting on with life. Nurses and doctors often make lousy patients.

I chose a recliner that allowed me to look out the window at the dreary, gray sky. How I thought that might cheer me up, I don't know. Snow began falling. People scampered across the street, coming out of the Ideal Market. I could almost taste croissant sandwiches of tomato, lettuce, onion, and avocado, washed down with orange juice. I savored the moment, knowing in a few hours nausea would drive all thoughts of food from my mind. Cars slowly wove down Broadway and I watched them, trying to keep my mind off Connie's starting an IV in my right hand. Like all the nurses I'd met in the oncology treatment area, she was kind and cheerful.

"HEY," a thin black woman hollered in the chair next to mine. "HEY! Whatcha doin' to me? You all pesterin' me all the time. I ain't done nothin' wrong. Why you stickin' that thing on me?" She grinned.

Connie smiled. "That's Miss Fester, Pam. She's been receiving treatments off and on for three years. She likes people to know she's here. She's a scream. She tries to make us feel guilty, but she loves us. She usually brings cookies. She's a wonderful woman and doesn't deserve the tough time she's had with her cancer exacerbations. I don't know how she keeps going. She told me once that hollering and complaining helps her tolerate her 'miserable treatments' easier. Some time ago, she noticed other patients laughing when they saw her smiling despite her complaints, so she's kept it up. She loves cheering up others. She's one in a million, so enjoy."

"HEY!" Miss Fester screamed. "Whatcha doin' with them scissors? Gonna cut my thumb off?"

Miss Fester's nurse said, "I'm adjusting your armband so you will be ready when the tech brings a unit of blood for you in a few minutes."

"BLOOD?" Miss Fester hollered. "I don't need no blood. If you all wouldn't take blood out of me every dang time I come in here, I wouldn't need no dang blood. All this fuss—can't even take a nap."

Miss Fester grinned at me. "Don't worry 'bout nothing, honey. These girls know what they'se doin'. Most of the time anyway." She gave her nurse the evil eye. "You like chocolate chip cookies, honey?" Miss Fester asked me. "There's some 'round here with your name on 'em. That is, if these nurses ain't eaten 'em all up already. They do like my cookies. You finished yet?" she demanded of her nurse. "I'd appreciate a little shut eye. Spent all morning bakin' them dang cookies. Would be nice to take a little nap while the vampire from the lab hooks me up to my dinner. Are you all servin' cocktails this afternoon? I sure could use one. HEY! Whatcha do-in' now?" she cried out as her nurse took two vials of blood. "I thought you all was puttin' some in, not takin' out more dang blood."

"We need to check blood counts for your doctor."

"ALWAYS wantin' somethin' from me," Miss Fester shouted, grinning like a Cheshire cat. "Can't do nothin' without somebody wantin' somethin' from me! Lord, have mercy!"

"IV's in," Connie told me. "Thanks to Miss Fester, I bet you didn't feel the pokes today. I blew the first one. Sorry. But we got a nice blood return on the second. I'll do the push drugs first, starting with Anzemet for your nausea. We either push that med or hang it with Decadron, but Dr. Sitarik told me we would not be giving Decadron today, right?"

"Right. And Miss Fester helped. That was the least painful IV yet."

I studied other patients while Connie pushed my drugs. A very pale, very emaciated young woman sat nearby. A young man's hand held hers. Not a single hair embellished her bald head, but a look of serenity graced her face—for a few minutes. A nurse slowly pushed a drug through the medication port in the woman's chest until a look of panic replaced the serenity.

"My throat is closing up," the patient croaked out, alarmed. "The surgical sutures in my neck feel like they're ripping apart."

The nurse relayed the concerns to Connie, who scooted off to confer with an oncologist, while the frightened patient remained in caring and competent hands. Within two minutes, Connie brought a filled syringe, and the drug was slowly pushed through the panic-stricken woman's port. As the drug took effect, she relaxed.

Within five minutes, she was laughing hysterically. "I feel so much better," she proclaimed.

"I'll have one of whatever she just got," I said.

"I pushed some Ativan to relax her muscles," Connie replied. "She'll feel okay for a while."

"Yeah," the patient responded, obviously hearing Connie. "I'm feeling A-OK! Yippee!"

A young family sat to my left. A man, in his early thirties, lay in a recliner while meds dripped through his IV. Two small children, about three and five years of age, bounced around him and the young woman sitting quietly by his side. Finally, the woman picked up the younger of the two girls and kissed her. She stood, kissed the man, and told him she would buy the girls a snack in the cafeteria. He adjusted the Broncos' ball cap, a recent souvenir of their second Super Bowl victory, on his bald head. The family was so young. At least my kids were older, and our primary bread-winner was healthy—so far. How frightening it must have been worrying about the future for him and his wife. I prayed God would protect them.

Connie hung my Cytoxan. "Okay, Pam. An hour and a half and you'll be out of here."

My husband showed up just before the Cytoxan ran out. "Thanks for picking me up, Bill."

"It would have been a long walk, Pam. I wasn't going to let my best girl trek home in this miserable weather."

Snow blanketed the ground and huge white flakes choked the sky. It was beautiful, but I imagined that blossoming flora and saplings would not fare well in this weather.

"We'll lose our flowers," I said wistfully.

"You know what this place needs?" Bill asked. "A sports bar. Yeah. A chemotherapy sports bar—belt down a drink while you lounge. What a concept."

"Except half the people here are too close to puking to drink alcohol," I challenged. "Except for Miss Fester. She wouldn't mind sidling up to the bar."

"Miss Fester?"

"That's me, honey child. I could go for a stiff one while I'm waitin' for this red goo to drip in. Want a cookie?" she asked as my nurse removed my IV.

Once Bill convinced me his trusty Jeep would have no trouble navigating the snowy streets, he and I dropped in at Barnes and Noble Booksellers. Snowplows had begun their runs down Pearl Street.

Bill and I haunted bookstores the way kids dawdled in toy stores. For years, our children bemoaned our inability to enter a mall without perusing the bookstores. It was a fault with which we could live. While Bill pored over computer manuals, I scrutinized the poetry stacks for W. B. Yeats, Seamus Heaney, and Patrick Kavanagh.

By the time we got home, I was extremely nauseous—my fault because I'd refused the Decadron. My head pounded and exhaustion consumed me within a couple of hours. Unable to concentrate on reading *The Playboy of the Western World* by J. M. Synge, I gave myself up to watching the movie, *A Simple Twist of Fate*. Afterwards, I collapsed in bed. At least without the Decadron, I'd sleep.

Chapter 25 - April 20th

Another Tuesday, and I did not want to be at work. The exhaustion I'd suffered since my treatment the Friday before had hardly waned. I'd dragged myself out of bed at 5:15 and lasted only eight minutes on my treadmill. I longed to crawl into bed—anybody's bed, and it was only a few minutes to eight. I'd have been willing to take a nap on an uncomfortable, body ache-producing exam table. I laid my head on my desk.

"Morning, Pam!" Dr. Hibbard yelled happily, sticking his head in my office. "Isn't it a beautiful day?"

"I really hadn't noticed, doc," I whimpered.

"You feeling okay?"

"I'm pooped, thank-you very much."

"You and Bill have a big weekend?"

"I had chemo on Friday, and although I spent the weekend in bed, it wasn't with Bill."

"You must be about finished with those treatments."

"One more to go. I thought having Monday off would revitalize me enough to get through the week, but I'm still tired. I'll get through it, but I am bone weary, to tell you the truth." The intercom paged me to Room 2. "Bring 'em on," I challenged.

I sensed reserve among the front desk staff as I walked past. Three more employees had submitted their resignations, citing personal reasons for leaving. We knew better, however. Discouragement over working perpetually short-staffed and being compensated with pitiful pay sent exhausted workers scurrying for new jobs. Like many health care facilities around the country saddled with responsibility for outlying clinics, Boulder Community Hospital faced a crisis. With poor insurance reimbursement, funds were sucked away in a spiraling whirlpool of debts.

Out of nine employees responsible for the efficient running of the office, the clinic stood to lose six within a two-month period. To add to the despair, our office manager, who was merely the most recent in a spate of managers, had decided to return to school for a master's degree in business and would be gone in two months. The family atmosphere generated by the close comradery of the clinic staff had disintegrated into an ugly divorce.

Everyone walked on eggshells. Tears flowed steadily, egos bruised easily, and control of frustrations was non-existent. Laughter that kept our spirits high was no longer heard. Whispered fragments of melancholic conversations pervaded the working spaces: the clinic was too small; the providers took too much time off; the hospital didn't care about employees at their distant clinics; the pay was abysmal; and staff members were tired of dealing with increasingly hostile patients who fought for too few appointment openings.

We desperately needed another provider and an office manager who wanted to manage. We needed more rooms, but there was nowhere to expand. The hospital vacillated between building a new clinic and moving us into one of the many office buildings under construction in Louisville. Believe me, we couldn't have cared less—we just needed more room. Until a decision was made, there would be no funds to update equipment or provide renovations for our deteriorating surroundings. While we waited for the powers above to render judgment, we drudged on with our limited emotional reserves and wondered aloud if we'd have a clinic at all with the current rash of resignations. Even the unflappable nursing staff had reached the end of their ability to cope.

"Why should the nurses worry about patients when the providers have lost interest?" Gail asked quietly. "At least it seems that way when two doctors are on vacation and a third one says, 'I *have* to have the same week off. Make it happen.' Do you have any idea how discouraged patients feel having to reschedule appointments, because their doctors decide to take off time at the last minute? Some of these patients schedule physicals months in advance. It isn't the doctor that gets yelled at—it's me, caught in the middle again. I can't blame the patients. I've just about had it, Pam." She sighed.

As have we all, I thought, opening the door to Room 2. I forced a smile for Mrs. Elizabeth Price, a seventy-two year old lady who had been a patient since the clinic first opened. I felt it a genuine honor to care for her. She was a fiercely independent, healthy woman who had no chronic problems and took no medications or supplements other than a handful of carefully selected vitamins.

"Morning, Mrs. Price. How can I help you today?"

"You can get rid of the pain in my back, that's what you can do for me," she snapped, but she had a twinkle in her eye.

"Feeling edgy this morning?"

"Yes, and you would, too, if you were in as much pain as I am."

"Tell me about it, Mrs. Price."

"Yesterday, a tingling and itching sensation started on the right side of my back, under my bra. I looked in the mirror but there wasn't anything there. This morning I noticed blisters."

"How about if I take a look after you change into one of these stylish patient gowns?"

"Suit yourself."

I stepped outside of the room while Mrs. Price removed her blouse and bra and put on a clinic gown. I thought about the last time I'd waited for Mrs. Price to change. Dr. Richards had been standing outside of Room 1, looking a bit flushed.

"Dr. Richard, are you okay?" I'd asked, concerned.

"Uh, Pam, I didn't see you there. I just had a very uncomfortable patient encounter."

"Do you want to talk about it?" I'd led him to an empty exam room.

"I'm scheduled to do a Pap on a twenty-three year old woman. I asked about her occupation, and she told me she works at Hooters. After we reviewed her medical and family history, I left the room for her to change. I distinctly remember telling her to leave the gown open in the back so she'd feel less exposed. When I walked back into the room, the patient whipped open her gown and said, 'What do you think, doctor? Are these great boobs or what?' "

"So, doc, what did you answer? Were they great hooters, er, breasts, or not?"

"As a matter of fact, they were great looking breasts. But that's beside the point. I don't think about a woman's breasts when I'm doing a physical. At least, I don't consciously do it. It's difficult maintaining professionalism when a patient pulls a stunt like that."

"You haven't told me how you responded to the patient's question?"

"I stammered, 'they're nice'. It was a bit awkward."

"She was just trying to get a rise out of you doc. You'll have to admit her come-on was a lot more direct than other female patients' lines you've encountered. May I assume your nurse will be standing by for the entire exam?"

"You'd better believe it," he said. He'd gotten through the rest of the exam, professional that he is.

And I was daydreaming again. Surely I'd given Mrs. Price enough time to change. When I opened the door, she said, "I thought you forgot all

210

about me, dear. And me thinking you didn't have to leave in the first place. I imagine I haven't got anything you haven't seen before."

"I wanted to give you some privacy while you changed, Mrs. Price."

"Why? You've seen it all when you've done my Paps."

"Mrs. Price, you are such a comedian. Let's take a look."

"Okay, let us. Although I think it will just be you looking and not us, unless you've got a midget standing behind you. And you're pretty short as it is."

"I prefer petit, thanks." I examined her back. "Just as I thought; you have herpes zoster."

"I don't have herpes!" Mrs. Price screamed. "I know where you get that stuff. And I've been a widow for twenty years."

"Mrs. Price, there are many forms of herpes and they're not all sexually transmitted. This is zoster—shingles. Have you ever heard of shingles?"

"My mom had it. Is that what's called a genetic disease?"

"No, ma'am, it's not. You had chickenpox as a child, right?"

"I did. Bad case, too. I had pox all over my body, including my ears, hair, and mouth. It was awful."

"Well, that chickenpox was caused by a virus. Although it didn't cause you any persistent problem, that virus attached itself to a nerve root. Now it's been reactivated."

"What caused a reactivation?"

"Lots of things can be implicated, like illness, stress..."

"Ah, ha! I knew that Billy would be the death of me. He's my grandson. He's sixteen and ran away from home last week. His parents are worried sick. They're camped at my house. The police have been over twice. Seems Billy and a friend may have broken into some homes in Longmont. We're all nervous wrecks." She reached up to scratch the painful area.

"Try not to scratch, Mrs. Price."

"It hurts and it itches. How do you know it's shingles?"

"If you look in the mirror tonight, you will notice fluid-filled blisters. They are arranged in a very specific pattern along the right side of your back, along what we call a dermatome. A dermatome is an area that is innervated by a specific nerve. In most cases, the chickenpox virus attaches to one nerve root, so you get a very distinctive, band-like pattern like yours."

"What am I going to do about this bra? It's killing me."

"You might leave your bra off until the lesions heal."

"And give young guys a thrill watching me jiggle?" she asked, snorting. "I don't think so."

"It's up to you, but that's what I'd do."

"Yeah, well you young girls think nothing of whipping out your boobies for any good looking male, but those of us who are older have to maintain some decency."

"I'm not exactly a young girl anymore."

"It depends on how you look at it, darling. So, how are you going to keep me from scratching myself to death?"

"I'm going to prescribe some prednisone that will help with the inflammation and itching, some hydrocodone for the pain, and some acyclovir to decrease viral replication and prevent some of the post-herpetic neuralgia."

"Say what?"

"Post-herpetic neuralgia. Sometimes pain can last for weeks or months after the lesions disappear. It doesn't happen too often, thank goodness, but studies have shown that medication can help prevent that complication."

"Terrific. Any more good news?"

"Nope. That's all. Knowing your past medical history, however, you will probably weather this just fine. Please call me if you have any problems. Oh, and don't be tooling around in your sports car while you're taking that pain medication."

"Great. Next you'll tell me to avoid my nightly couple of beers. Is this contagious? I know chickenpox was."

"Avoid the beer if you're taking hydrocodone for pain. And no, this isn't contagious in the same sense that chickenpox was. Chickenpox is a respiratory illness. The virus spreads by coughing and talking. Shingles spreads if someone touches a broken blister. The virus is present in the blister. The person wouldn't develop shingles, but chickenpox, if he or she was never exposed to it. Keep the lesions covered until they're all scabbed over. Got it?"

"If I cover the blisters until they scab up, no one will catch this from me. Is that right?"

"You've got it. Any other questions?"

"No. I'll take my prescriptions and get out of here. By the way, it's been hell trying to get an appointment with you. Have you been on vacation or something like that?"

"Definitely something like that. You have a great day. I always enjoy seeing you."

"Well, maybe next time we can just visit at the grocery store. I don't much enjoy coming to the doctor's office. I could catch something."

"You could, indeed," I laughed.

As I left the room, I almost ran into Jen, one of our medical assistants. "I'm your slave today, Pam," she said, handing me a Q-tip and a cup with liquid nitrogen in it.

"Am I to assume my next patient has plantar warts?"

"Ooh. Give the nurse practitioner a cigar. You've got two patients in the room. Don has warts and his sister Angie has acne. She wants a derm referral."

The kids were impressed with the steaming cup of liquid nitrogen I used to treat a dozen warts on the bottoms of Don's feet. They were even more impressed when I poured the unused solution on the carpet. The liquid nitrogen immediately evaporated, forming a cloud of smoke. I turned to Angie. She had facial pustules and blackheads—no cystic acne. With little difficulty, I convinced Angie we could provide care for her.

Jen grabbed me as I left the room. "Your next patient won't be so quick a visit. I have a positive pregnancy test in my hand and a seventeen-year-old girl who has been on birth control pills for two years."

"Not a great combination. I assume she is not happy."

"Not unless those are tears of joy."

"Is anyone with her?"

"She brought a girlfriend."

I closed the door and sat across from a young girl with red-rimmed eyes.

"It's positive, isn't it?" Her eyes pleaded for disagreement.

"Do you want to discuss this in front of your friend, Missy? Or would you prefer she wait out front?"

"Beth's my best friend. You can say anything in front of her."

I took a deep breath. "It's positive, Missy."

"Oh, God, oh God! How could this happen? I didn't miss any pills."

"The pill isn't one hundred per cent effective. It's close, but pregnancy can occasionally occur. When did your last period start?"

"The end of February. I didn't have a period last month, but I knew I couldn't be pregnant. I took every pill on time."

"Were you on any antibiotics since your last period, Missy?"

"Uh huh, the first three weeks in March. I went to the urgent care a couple of times, because I had a bad sinus infection."

"Did you mention you were on birth control pills?"

"No. I don't consider them medication."

"Missy, has anyone ever mentioned that some antibiotics make the pill less effective?"

"No, I wasn't told that."

"Condoms need to be used as back-up to your birth control pills when you take antibiotics. Do you encourage your boyfriend to use condoms?"

She shook her head.

"It's possible that the antibiotics contributed to your becoming pregnant. There's no way to know for sure. At your age, condoms are always a good idea. They help prevent sexually transmitted diseases."

"I've been with the same guy for six months, and he told me he was clean."

"Have you noticed any change in vaginal discharge lately?"

"Yeah, it smells bad."

"I'd like to check you today for infection. Do you have any abdominal pain?"

"No."

"Missy, I have a suspicion you knew this test would be positive."

"Uh huh."

"Do you know what your options are?"

"Uh huh."

"Have you decided what you want to do?"

"I'm going to have an abortion. No way am I ready for this."

I bit my lip to stop from saying something I knew I'd regret later—something that would not help the situation. "Have you considered having the baby and allowing a loving couple to adopt it?"

"I'm not going to let some brat ruin my senior year," she spat out venomously.

I took a deep breath. "I know you don't know me, so you may not feel comfortable discussing this with me, but can you talk to your mother?"

"Yeah. She's way cool. I was born when she was fifteen."

"Please talk to her soon. If you decide to keep the baby, you will need a referral to an obstetrician. I can do that for you. Do you have any questions for me?"

"I don't think so. I've got a lot to think about."

"And not too long to think. Options diminish as the weeks go by."

"I know."

"Please call me if you have questions. I'll phone you in a couple of days to see how you've fared with your mother." I handed Missy a business card and added my home phone number. I didn't give out my home number often, but I occasionally felt it justified, especially when the subject might prove difficult or embarrassing to discuss with "yet another person" like the on-call doc. "I'll be glad to talk to you any time, Missy. I'm going to step outside so you can undress."

As I waited outside the door, Dr. Richard invaded my thoughts again. I'd been employed at the clinic only a few months when I'd faced a similar situation requiring counseling about pregnancy options.

"Do you have a minute, Dr. Richard?" I'd asked.

He'd led me into the kitchen. "What's bothering you, Pam?"

"Dr. Richard, we're both Catholic. Even though I would never impose my beliefs on a patient, I torment myself when a woman doesn't want to continue her pregnancy. How do you deal with it?"

"I don't torture myself, because the choice isn't ours to make, Pam. All we can do is apprise women of their options, make sure they know we're available for questions, and encourage them to seek professional help no matter what the decision. Beyond that, our hands are tied."

"You're right. I know we're here to serve others, and I'm not one for proselytizing generally, but I feel so helpless. This is such a huge decision, a life impacting decision—and I'm not just talking about one life."

"Pam," he'd said, giving me a hug, "just make sure they know you're available if needed. That's all you can do. You stay up nights worrying about these patients, don't you?"

"I do. Thanks for listening."

"I didn't help much."

"You did, doc. I appreciate it."

After Missy left, I walked back to my office with the intention of working on charts. Instead of sitting at the desk, however, I stood at the window thinking about Missy and her baby. The sky clouded over. It had been sunny when I came to work, but now the sky looked as dismal as my heart felt. I hated how often the job emotionally traumatized me. I managed to get through four patient charts before I was summoned to see my next patient. Thinking about Missy instead of paying attention, I caught my shoe on a torn piece of carpet and ungracefully landed on my knees.

Dr. Pittenger helped me up. "Have a nice trip, Pam?"

"I did. I had my mind on a patient."

"It would be nice if someone would either move us or fix this clinic so we wouldn't have to think about what we're doing." She chuckled and walked away.

I limped to Room 2 and picked up the chart. The chief complaint was a sore throat. After Missy, I was ready for a case that would be less gut wrenching. As I laid the chart on the desk however, I noticed angry bruises on Margie Brendon's face and a swollen black eye. The purplish outline of fingers and a thumb encircling her left arm were clear evidence that a sore throat was the least of this woman's problems.

"Mrs. Brendon, I'm Pam Stockho, the nurse practitioner here. How can I help you today?"

"I have a sore throat. I want to make sure I don't have strep."

"I can help you with that, but I'm concerned about the bruises on your face and arm. Will you tell me about them?"

Margie Brendon cried. "I fell down some stairs. That's all."

"Did that fall include someone grabbing your arm?" I touched the woman's hand.

"He didn't mean to do it. It was my fault. I was supposed to be home by half past seven, and I didn't get home until after eight. He was worried."

"Has he hit you before?"

"Only if I deserved it. It was my fault. I love him. He promised he won't hit me again. He said he was sorry."

"How many times has he promised he wouldn't hit you again, Mrs. Brendon?"

She sobbed.

"Mrs. Brendon, checking for strep is easy. But your bruises worry me. I have to report this to the police. Please speak to a police officer today."

"No! I won't go to the police. I won't press charges. It was an accident. Please don't say anything!"

"The law requires me to report this, Mrs. Brendon. No one deserves to be hit. I'll give you the number of the Boulder County Safehouse in Lafayette, and I advise you to go there."

"No! You can't make me. I can do whatever I want. I'm not going to let you examine me. You can go to hell, for all I care!" She stood up, walked out, and slammed the door.

The door opened cautiously. "Pam, are you in here?" Jen asked. I covered my face with my hands. "Are you okay?"

"No, I'm not okay. This is the kind of day that makes me hate this job. I feel completely useless. I'm so upset I could cry. God, help me."

"Pam," Jen said, sitting beside me, "we've all admired you during these last few months. Sometimes we wonder how you keep going despite your tiredness. Most patients enjoy seeing you, but you can't solve everyone's problems. Please don't take these failures so personally."

I looked up. "Life is unbearable for so many. People face decisions that affect their whole lives—will determine if they have a life at all. I wish I had the wisdom to choose words more carefully, so patients might be more open to suggestion."

"Suggestions are all you can offer, Pam. They make the choices. You aren't God. You have to accept you've done your best."

"You sound like Dr. Richard." I stood. "Is my next patient here?"

"She just arrived. Give me a minute before going to Room 1."

The rest of the morning was uneventful, giving me time to regroup and ask God's help to say the right things, to bring comfort instead of increasing stress. There were so many jobs that required little emotional expenditure. What had I been thinking entering a profession that sapped so much emotional and physical energy? Why put myself through that day after day? The answer was simply that I loved what I did. Situations in which I found myself emotionally vulnerable often resulted in great personal satisfaction, because I helped another human being—perhaps made a small difference in his or her day. And truthfully, I'd not had as awful a morning as this one in a long time. I gathered my last few patients' charts and headed for my office, hoping to catch up on paperwork during lunch.

As I eased into my chair, Jen popped her head around the corner. "I have a work-in for you, Pam. The fellow is complaining of left knee pain. I think he's drunk. He sure smells like it."

"Thank-you, Jen. Remind me to cross you off my Christmas list this year." I stood up, grabbed my stethoscope, and headed to Room 2.

"Just follow your nose, Pam."

God, give me strength. I grabbed the patient's chart. He'd been asked to update his patient information. Unlike his previous information form, the form he completed today was all but illegible. His signature was a wavy line. I opened the door. The man was weaving unsteadily, bracing himself against the exam table. The smell of alcohol oozed from every pore.

"Mr. Simpson, why don't you sit down while we discuss your problem? You seem unsteady."

"Sssnothing wrong with my feet," he said, looking down at them. He weaved unsteadily.

I grabbed his arm and guided him into a chair. He stared at me with red, glazed eyes.

"What can I do for you today, Mr. Simpson?"

"Give me some fucking pain meds for my fucking knee."

"What happened?"

"I fucking fell. Whas it to you?"

I attempted to examine his knee, but he batted my hand away. "That fucking hurts!"

"Where does it hurt, Mr. Simpson?" I tried, with increasing difficulty, to control my temper.

"Whole thing. Just want sssomething for pain."

"Mr. Simpson, how much have you had to drink today?"

"Few beers, s'all. My knee fucking hurts. Beers help."

"Did you drive to the clinic today?"

"Yeah. Whas it to you?"

"You shouldn't be driving in your condition. You've had too much to drink."

"Not drunk; few beers—s'all."

"Mr. Simpson, I will X-ray your knee to make sure you don't have a fracture, since you won't let me examine you. I'll provide a brace for your knee, if nothing's broken, and I will call for a taxi to take you home. I will even pay for it. I'll recheck you in a day or two. However, I will not give you narcotics for pain, because you have been drinking. If you drive your car out of our parking lot today, I will call the police. Our radiology tech will come for you in a few minutes to X-ray your knee." So much for my compassion!

Within four minutes, Krystal was in my office. "X-rays done already?" I inquired.

"He left. He told me to tell you that you were a "fucking bitch" and walked out. Here's his chart."

I called the Louisville Police Department and reported a drunk driver. "Did you get a copy of his driver's license?"

"No, we did not."

"Then there is nothing we can do," the police officer responded.

"You mean to tell me you are going to let an inebriated individual drive on the streets of Louisville?"

"That's right, ma'am. Without a copy of his driver's license, there is nothing we can do."

"Until he kills someone," I thought sadly, hanging up the phone. I probably should have called back to verify what I'd been told was police policy, but I didn't. By that time, I was too angry.

I retrieved my salad from the refrigerator and was settled in my office when Krystal walked in. "Pam, do your kids know anyone at Columbine High School?"

"I don't think so. Why?"

"The television is on in the waiting room. The police have staked out the school. Guns have been fired inside the school. Kids are running out the doors, saying students have been shot."

"Oh, my God!" I jumped up and rammed my left knee against the desk. I limped out to the waiting room to hear an announcer say, "...and at this time, the exact number of dead and injured inside the school is unknown. The estimate thus far is as high as twenty-five dead." The cameraman panned the school as dozens of students ran out of doors.

...

Twenty-four hours later, newspaper headlines screamed that twelve students and one teacher had been brutally murdered, and about twenty more students were injured. The two gunmen were dead, and fifteen families grieved. The state of Colorado and the entire nation shared their torment. I read the stories associated with the shootings at Columbine with a mixture of anguish and anger. Although both my father and husband were career military men, I never permitted guns in my home. Bill still occasionally reminded me of the day I forced him to sell the Winchester rifle he'd had for years.

I'd never forgotten the mental image of a fourteen-year-old boy coding as paramedics brought him into the ER where I worked in Virginia. CPR was begun and a chest tube inserted into his right chest where the bullet lodged. He'd been cleaning his father's gun when it discharged. He was so young. I begged the ER doctor to keep working on him.

"We've tried for over half an hour, Pam. He's gone. There's nothing more we can do."

"He's only fourteen," I said. "He's someone's son. He's only fourteen." My son, Jon, had just turned fourteen.

After Columbine, newspapers around the world condemned Americans' easy access to guns. I couldn't argue with their disapproval, but the sorrow I felt was echoed by everyone I knew—regardless of whether or not they approved of guns in the home.

Two boys died of self-inflicted wounds, but their possession of weapons was not the whole story. They were outcasts, bullied by those who thought themselves superior. I could never condone or understand what they did, but to me it symbolized a world replete with examples of oppression and injustice toward one group by another.

On a broader scale than Columbine, the people of Kosovo were in the news, because they had long suffered unspeakable brutality. Why, I mused, couldn't we all get along? Why waste life being consumed with hate when so much good could be done with the same energy? Why couldn't those who squandered resources terrorizing and abusing others turn those same monies into improving the lives of the poor? Why couldn't we appreciate and celebrate differences—be it race, religion, gender, sexual orientation, or physical challenge? Differences made life interesting.

I thanked God every day that those of us who searched for good in others outnumbered those who looked for faults. Wouldn't it be grand if we pointed out something positive every time we met another person? I knew that positive self-esteem stemmed from much more than a few kind remarks, but each bit helped.

I'll not deny that we Americans have been, and continue to be, guilty of persecuting others. Stupidity self-perpetuates. I have witnessed events that led me to question what century I lived in. Inconceivably, I saw a Ku Klux Klan march sometime in either 1996 or 1997, when I visited home in North Carolina. I had attended Mass in Hope Mills only to find my exit barred by hordes of hooded jackasses marching down Hope Mills Road.

The thought that such demonstrations are legal makes me want to vomit. Freedom of speech might be a Constitution-granted privilege in this country, but I can't understand why such freedom allows denigration of anyone. Believe me, I have more than my share of faults, but I try my best to accept and embrace others. And yeah, I'll admit I sometimes fall short of that lofty goal.

Chapter 26 - April 28th

I stared at the ceiling, as I'd done for nearly an hour. I couldn't drag myself out of bed. I rolled over and stared at the clock—almost ten a.m. Surely that was wrong. I felt too tired for it to be that late. I willed myself to think about projects I'd completed, trying, I suppose, to convince myself I'd made good use of my weeks at home. Ironically, I could work when I felt terrible, those first few days after treatments. It was the week I enjoyed a little more energy, but a depleted white blood cell count, that kept me chained to the house. The increase in energy I felt the second week of my three-week cycles was miles away from the vigor I'd enjoyed before starting chemotherapy. Exhaustion followed me through each day, and I often wondered if I'd ever come close to regaining the stamina I'd once taken for granted.

When I felt able, I busied myself with cleaning the house and compiling more photo albums for the kids. I edited and copied cassette tapes we'd sent Bill during the years he'd been at sea. I hoped the children would enjoy hearing the stories and messages we'd sent Daddy. Typical was Jon, aged two-and-a-half, demanding of Bill (whose voice was wafting airily from a cassette): "Stop talking, Daddy! I'm talking to you! How did Daddy fit in that box, Mommy?"

Sharing pictures and tapes with the children helped me rekindle the love for Bill that had waned through the years. Emotionally, we had grown stronger after each hardship we'd endured—the six-month separations, the frequent moves. But they were also the times that drove an emotional wedge between us, because Bill was rarely around when the household goods were packed and the children cried for toys that might not be seen for weeks. He was home only once when the boxes were unloaded from the moving van. I usually waded through them alone, trying to set up a new home with three small children demanding every moment of my waking hours.

Demanded was too harsh, because I loved being needed. I adored sharing walks, pets' escapades, outings to parks, rides to McDonald's, movies, and books with them. But it was exhausting. Homecoming, when the sub pulled into port, sometimes months after we'd moved, was welcome—it always was, but my simmering cauldron of resentment at being a single parent and putting my little ones through yet another move every three years grew over the years. The children made friends only to have to tearfully bid them goodbye two or three years later—as did I.

Pulling up stakes wasn't entirely depressing, of course. We explored new ports. The submarine force was relatively small compared to the rest of the Navy. Moves invariably brought renewed friendships and exciting new experiences.

I stared at the ceiling again and felt totally unmotivated. It was the middle of my week off, and all I wanted to do was sleep.

The night before, I had written: "start writing again" at the top of my to-do list, but I wasn't sure I could face my stupid computer yet. It hated me. No one could convince me it didn't have a mind of its own. My commands were laughed at. It taunted me, daring me to press a button so it could erase hours of work. Maybe I'd put off writing until tomorrow. Today, I'd just lie in bed.

Heidi had other ideas. Bill let the dogs out, but I was responsible for their breakfast. Heidi stood on my chest, slobbering on my face, her eyes insistent that I move my sorry butt. Hannah and Holly barked. My reverie was at an end.

After they ate, I harnessed the three dogs and made my way to the walking trail that wound behind the houses perched on the edge of the hill across the street. In spite of my depleted energy, I knew a walk would get my heart racing, my epinephrine pumping, and invigorate me—either that or kill me.

The dogs, excited to escape the house, dragged me down the street. They'd never been to obedience school. I taught them to sit, stay, eat, sleep, and poop, but that's about it, so I couldn't complain when they pulled me, hell-bent for the resident prairie dogs that lived on the hillside. As they ran for their burrows, the furry little critters returned my dogs' barks.

I enjoyed flashes of bright flowers as I raced by, but my feet barely hit the pavement. My favorite yard was on the west end of the walkway, and thankfully my pets were usually pooped by the time we reached it. There was little color, save a few scattered sunflowers in the summer, but gracing the yard on tiered earth were a dozen headstones, headless angel figures, crosses, and urns. The macabre sight reminded me of all the cemeteries I'd loved through the years, but as much as I enjoyed strolling through grave-yards, I doubted I'd ever create one in my backyard. I always expected Gomez Addams to pop out the back door of the house, but he never did.

The dogs panted as they reached the steep incline that would lead back to our house. They weren't the only ones panting. Little would be accomplished during the rest of my day.

After we arrived home, I filled the girls' water dishes. They collapsed on the floor, panting. I grabbed a biography of the Irish writer, Brendan Behan, and gracelessly sprawled across a chair. The dogs and I could vegetate for a couple of hours before I faced my sadistic computer.

By the time I finished reading about Behan's stints in prison, I craved a bit of cheer. I sorted through the mail and read a couple of letters from friends living on the East Coast. Although I'd spared casual friends my pathetic tale of woe, I'd written to close friends, and I'd received many notes of encouragement. After reading my letters, I felt ready to *offer* some support. I called Mrs. Lieberman, the wife of my patient with testicular cancer.

"Stan's back in the hospital," she said.

"I'm sorry. What happened, Mrs. Lieberman?"

"After Stan visited you in the office, we saw the urologist together. As you know, the urologist confirmed your suspicion of cancer. Stan was operated on the same night. He's trying to keep his sense of humor; his new e-mail moniker is something like *YeOldeOneNut*. After surgery, everything looked fine. A CAT scan failed to show any masses or suspicious lesions anywhere else. Stan felt pretty good until last week, when he complained of back pain. Dr. Bachelder thought he might have pulled a muscle. Two days ago, he began dragging his left leg when he walked, and yesterday he could barely move. Dr. Bachelder rechecked him yesterday afternoon and ordered an MRI of the lumbar spine. It showed a mass. The oncologist thinks his testicular cancer metastasized to his lower back. Only about three percent of patients with testicular cancer suffer metastasis to the spine. It figures it would happen to us. What's the saying? If we didn't have bad luck, we'd have no luck at all.

"The mass in his spine wasn't apparent on the original CAT scan, and the radiologist mentioned that if he hadn't known where to look because of Stan's symptoms, he might have missed it on the MRI. Stan had surgery on his spine last night. I'm exhausted, but I shouldn't complain. Stan is going through so much. They're telling him he may never walk or have bladder control again." She sobbed.

My chest tightened. "Mrs. Lieberman, I'm sorry." I said nothing more until she stopped crying. "Do you have any help preparing meals?"

"Volunteers from our church have brought food. I'm very thankful. Between visits to the hospital and working, I have little reserve."

"You're working through this?"

"It keeps my mind from thinking about the future, but I may take extended leave. Stan will require a lot of help for a while—maybe forever. It's so hard to think of my thirty-four year old husband as an invalid." She cried again. I waited. "The oncologist talked to us about chemotherapy today, Pam. I was so disappointed. It's a difficult treatment regimen. Each cycle will be three weeks, but he'll have to endure chemotherapy five days a week for one week, then one day each of the other two weeks. I don't know how I'll manage. I certainly can't work when he has chemotherapy five days a week."

"I'm sorry, Mrs. Lieberman. I truly am. Treatment regimens differ depending on age, type of cancer, and prognosis. One of the girls at work mentioned her sister-in-law has breast cancer and that she's been told she would be bald before the end of chemotherapy. Since I haven't lost all my hair, my co-worker was going to suggest her sister-in-law get a second opinion, until I mentioned therapies may vary greatly, even if two patients suffer the same general diagnosis. Her sister-in-law will be receiving the drug Adriamycin, so she will lose her hair. It's all very confusing."

"I'm certainly learning more than I want to about cancer treatments, Pam. God forgive me, but it helped to leave the hospital for a few hours. I have to be strong for Stan, but I'm falling apart inside."

Knowing she had two teen-aged boys, I asked, "How are your children doing?"

"They appear to be weathering this better than I am. Teens figure they're going to live forever, so they imagine Stan will too. I hope they're right."

"I hope so too."

"Pam, may I ask you a question?"

"Of course, Mrs. Lieberman."

"Please call me Sheila."

"Sheila. What would you like to ask?"

"I've been learning about testicular cancer. I've read that if it's caught early, it's pretty easy to treat; Stan is having these problems, because he waited too long to be checked. Is that right?"

I forced out a deep breath. I hated *what if* questions. What if I'd paid closer attention? What if I'd checked myself regularly? What if I'd been rechecked as the doctor asked? It was true that if men checked their testicles every month and came in quickly after finding a mass, treatment was easier and metastasis less likely. A prognosis like Stan's often came from waiting, but there were few absolutes when dealing with cancer. Even when one knew the right path, denial played a powerful role. My answer was too long in coming.

"Pam? Are you there?"

"Sorry, Sheila. I was thinking about your question."

"It's true, isn't it? If he'd come in earlier, he might not be facing all this."

"He might not. But human nature what it is, none of us makes the best choices all the time."

"That's true. Pam, do you see patients for sports physicals?"

"I do."

"If I send my boys to you for their physicals, would you teach them to do testicular exams?"

"How old are they?"

"Fifteen and seventeen."

"I will. Please let them know they'll be seeing a woman, though. Some guys about that age are shy."

"I'll let them know, Pam."

"If they'd feel more comfortable being checked by a male, I know either Dr. Hibbard or Dr. Richard would explain the procedure to your boys."

"Thanks. That lifts one concern from my burdened mind. I'd better get back to the hospital, but I appreciate your call. I'll stop into the clinic in a few days to say, 'Hi'."

"I'd like that, thanks. Take care of yourself, Sheila. Please let me know if I can help you."

"I will. Thank-you. I'll talk to you later."

...

I'd barely replaced the receiver when Lisa rang. "How's it going, Pam?"

"I'm fine."

"You don't sound fine."

"I'm tired. That's all. And I'm still nauseated a week and a half after my last treatment. I'm alternating between hot flashes and cold chills."

"Either you're going through menopause or have a bad bug."

"Unfortunately, I think it's the former. Hey, does that mean I have the right to be bitchy now? Can I pass it off on menopause?"

"I don't think so. The girls at work won't buy it. You've been bitchy too long already." She chuckled.

"Nice, Lisa. Very nice."

"You're not feeling as bad as you did last week, Pam?"

"No. I'm better."

"That's good. You were looking pretty pale, lady. And I was worried about all the dizziness you were having. You seemed to be in the bathroom a lot."

"Thanks for noticing my frequent treks to the toilet. If it wasn't urinary frequency, it was diarrhea—all in all a terrific week."

"I don't know how you kept up with your patients, Pam."

"Ah, thinking about others' problems kept my mind off mine."

"Except when you hogged the bathroom."

"Except then. I take it you miss me, although there's more bathroom time for everyone else."

"Believe it or not, we miss you a lot, but I shouldn't tell you that. You'll get a swelled head."

"Not to worry. I'm experiencing some swelling, but it isn't my head. Have you been busy?"

"It's crazy here. I'll have you know I'm sacrificing part of my lunch break to talk to you."

"I'm deeply moved."

"You should be. Anyway, the place is in chaos. This morning, Dr. Richard called in sick at ten minutes to eight, so the front desk scurried to re-schedule his appointments. His eight and eight-fifteen a.m. appointments were worked in with Dr. Bachelder and Dr. Pittenger. They were both fully booked before the clinic opened. Eighteen patients who called before nine o'clock had to be seen today, so the two docs were seriously overbooked. It was a huge mess. It's chronically like that now. We need another full-time doctor or nurse practitioner, but there's no space. And we couldn't get a substitute provider today."

"I wish I could have come to work."

"Don't worry about it. We'll get by. Besides, since I'm in the back, I am pretty protected from the turmoil around the nurse's station."

"How about the new clinic the hospital promised to build for us?"

"The hospital scrapped the new building idea. They were relying on recruiting a group of surgeons to operate a day surgery unit to make it a profitable venture. When that plan fell through, the hospital decided to re-view other options for us."

"The hospital already owns the land, and we desperately need more space, Lisa. How much longer do they expect us to operate in such cramped quarters? We're going to lose patients and more staff, if not the doctors themselves, if we don't make changes."

"The patients are really frustrated not being able to get same day appointments, that's for sure," said Lisa. "We're still able to work-in emer-gencies, but patients needing routine appointments may wait several days. The doctors' physicals and Paps are booked until the beginning of August. Everyone is exasperated. The staff has had it. You know about the rash of employee resignations."

"God, it's awful, Lisa." And I would be sitting on my derriere for another five days before receiving a blessing to return to work. "We'll be lucky if we can keep the clinic running. I'll be honest, Lisa. If I didn't have to deal with cancer, I might be looking for another job. I don't mind working hard, but the stress of working at that crazy clinic is beginning to affect my patient care. When does the hospital anticipate our moving?"

"They're weighing options now. The city's building code won't allow expansion of our present facility, and no one, save Dr. Hibbard, wants to do that anyway. The present layout wouldn't work even if we could enlarge the building—the front desk is too small, the nurse's station is tiny, and some of the exam rooms are hardly bigger than closets. We need more office space. People are beginning to talk about what you and Dr. Richard do in your office."

"Are they?"

"Yes. We're so desperate for comic relief that we're starting rumors to lighten the tension. How about lunch tomorrow at the Mason Jar?"

"I'd love it, although I'm not sure that your regaling me with stories about the clinic will help my lunch digest."

"Forget the clinic. You can tell me what you've been reading about Ireland. How is your writing coming along?"

I gagged. She heard me. "All this time off, and you're not writing? This is your big chance."

"I know. I know. I'm trying to get a mind set."

"Mind set? Just sit down and write."

"It's not that easy, Lisa. I love writing, but psyching myself up to sit down to that blasted computer is tough."

"You can do it. I know you can."

"Grrr!"

"See you tomorrow. I'll pick you up at noon, Pam."

I hung up the phone and massaged my left arm for a few minutes. The numbness along the back of my upper arm, axilla, and lateral breast was waning slowly, replaced by intermittent pains so sharp I occasionally gasped. There was persistent burning in those areas. I was weathering the recovery of nerves awakening from the surgeries I'd had, but the pain was often intense. Even more aggravating was a constant itchy feeling in my upper arm that no amount of rubbing or scratching sated.

I dragged out my laptop and stared at it. How difficult could this be? I asked myself. I turned it on and punched up Microsoft Word. There, facing me, was a big blank white screen. Not one intelligent thought crossed my mind.

Chapter 27 - May 7th

The next week and a half flew by as I engrossed myself in work and writing. Well, okay, I sat in front of my laptop until random thoughts floated by. My short-term memory became affected by the chemotherapy and my distress over it consumed me. I'd read about that possible side effect and hoped it would pass me by, but fleeting thoughts plagued me on a regular basis. At first, I failed to remember grocery items I'd thought of needing only moments earlier. The kids chalked it up to Alzheimer's. I preferred to think of it as cerebral clutter or brain farts. But unfortunately, the symptoms worsened rapidly, so I resorted to keeping lists. It hadn't affected my patient care much, although occasionally I'd begin writing a prescription and sit like an idiot until the elusive drug popped into my pathetic brain. What a frustration!

I faced my greatest challenge writing. It seemed ironic that I finally had time to pursue my dream of writing when my brain teased me with intermittent farts of recollection. I knew exactly what I wanted to write. Sentences floated ethereally through my consciousness, but before I could grasp them and spit out the words, they would evaporate. I pictured the ordered convolutions of my cerebrum replaced by cheesecloth; little words slipped through the holes and drove me crazy on a regular basis.

I'd conjure up every malapropism even remotely close to a particular word, trying to resurrect an entire sentence by grasping for that pivotal combination of letters, but the word I sought usually escaped my quest until I opened my thesaurus and pored through it. That and my dictionaries became my closest friends—actually, not bad company to keep.

I slowly came to the realization that if nursing didn't work out, I'd never be a quick-witted talk show host or paid lecturer. I prayed my problem would vanish, but studies I read indicated patients still experienced short-term memory loss secondary to chemotherapy up to eight to ten years after treatment. Terrific! But on the other hand, the thought that I might have eight to ten years to test those conclusions brought me great comfort.

Although I bemoaned my losses, I soon found reason to celebrate. The day of my last treatment arrived. I walked on air as I waited for Dr. Sitarik. This was it; this was the last one! I still faced radiation treatments, but the side effects, I'd been told, were minimal compared to chemotherapy: a little skin redness, some pain, more fatigue. I hoped chemotherapy had wiped out most of the rapidly dividing cancer cells that had migrated to body parts unknown. With the increasing side effects of the last few weeks, I knew chemotherapy had destroyed a lot of rapidly dividing normal cells.

I prayed a lot. God and I'd had a pretty good relationship for years, but now I talked to him more like a friend. I occasionally postulated I was becoming psychotic, but since I didn't answer myself, mutter in public, or receive any personal revelations from the Almighty, I imagined my sanity remained relatively intact.

While I waited for Dr. Sitarik, I stood at the third story window overlooking my little part of the world. The Flatirons teased me in the distance. Although it was nearly the middle of May, and Mother's Day lurked two days in the future, mountain peaks within view of my beloved Flatirons remained snowcapped and would remain so until the end of July or August. By the third week in September, the area would receive its first snowfall, and the mountains would be dressed again in white until the following summer.

I watched people dart in and out of the Masa Grill, Noodles and Company, and the Ideal Market at the strip mall across the street. I was fast becoming a voyeur. Everyone seemed in such a hurry. I closed my eyes. Once upon a time, I had been in a rush. No more.

A car honking, followed by a crash, riveted my eyes to the parking lot. Two cars, approaching the same parking spot from opposite directions, had collided. The drivers exited their vehicles angrily, slamming doors. One man pushed at the other. A boxing match ensued. Within four minutes, two police cars pulled up, and officers pulled the men apart. The damage to the cars didn't look half as bad as the damage to the men's faces. There was another honk as a blue SUV pulled in front of a car on Broadway, narrowly missing the car's front bumper. The SUV's driver shot his hand out of the driver's window and extended his middle finger. The car's driver slammed on the brakes and the horn. I turned from the window as the door opened.

Dr. Sitarik read my chart as he walked toward me. "Your white cell count today is only 2.8. That's a little low to hit you with another treatment today."

A crushing sensation shot through my chest as I realized he might not let me complete my therapy today. Please, God, let me finish this today. Please!

Dr. Sitarik looked at my crestfallen face. I'd said nothing. He continued. "If this were any treatment other than the last one, I would have you wait a couple of weeks to provide time for your immune system to recover. Since this will be your final treatment, I will allow you to proceed as long as your exam is normal."

I let out the breath I'd been holding. Dr. Sitarik continued talking, but I'd not been listening. "I'm sorry. I missed what you were saying."

"I wondered if you've had any new side effects."

"No—about the same as last time, except I'm more tired. I've had fewer mouth ulcers. My hair is thinning like crazy, but at least I still have some. Otherwise, I'm okay. My attitude is better—I'm sure it has nothing to do with the fact that today will be my last treatment."

He left while I changed; then, he checked my breasts, felt for enlarged lymph nodes, listened to my heart and lungs, and palpated my abdomen.

"Everything seems fine," he said. "We'll recheck your white count in three weeks and then talk about scheduling radiation treatments." He extended his hand to say goodbye. "You've weathered your treatments well. I have no doubt your recent weight loss and regular exercise program contributed to maintaining your stamina. Keep it up."

"Thanks, Doctor Sitarik."

Trepidation overtook me as I walked to the treatment area. After today, I'd no longer have the security of regular chemotherapy to combat my cancer. Yup, I was really going to miss having poisons drip through my vein. I'd probably pine for side effects. I managed a smile for Patty as I sat down. Somehow it seemed appropriate that my nurse today would be the caring woman who'd helped me through the majority of my treatments.

"Hi, Pam. You're the first customer this afternoon." She reviewed the doctor's orders and pulled prescription medications, already mixed in their syringes, from their respective drawers.

"Which means you probably had a very busy morning, Patty."

"It was very busy. The weather is so gorgeous, everyone came in early so they'd have a few hours to enjoy being outside."

I wondered how many patients would truly enjoy the weather *after* chemotherapy, but I said nothing. Patty expertly inserted a 24-gauge needle into my right hand and began pushing medications. I watched people scamper across the street. Tow trucks removed the two disabled vehicles while ambulance staff examined the recalcitrant drivers. The bloodied men still appeared angry and intermittently raised clenched fists at each other.

I watched in amusement as someone pulled in and out of a parking space half a dozen times to align a car. Emerging from the vehicle, a tiny, elderly lady, barely taller than her automobile, seemed oblivious to the ambulance and police cars, which were parked only a few yards away. When the woman finally noticed their flashing lights, she dropped her purse. She picked up her bag and shuffled toward the grocery store, walking directly in the path of a car. The driver narrowly missed hitting her.

I adored Boulder, but some residents drove me crazy. They crossed against traffic, against signs lit up with "don't walk", with complete disregard for anyone else on the planet. Worst were the bicyclists who assumed traffic laws were meant for anyone but themselves. Not infrequently I, obeying the speed laws and traffic lights, slammed on my brakes as a bicyclist cut in front of my car. My heroic efforts to prevent maiming were often rewarded with nasty looks or obscene gestures, probably because I had the audacity to drive a car in the first place. Rob dubbed these unthinking, self-absorbed walkers and bicyclists *pestrians*. Thankfully, *pestrians* made up an irritating minority of Boulderites.

I drank in the room I would hopefully be seeing for the last time. Over the next hour and a half, while my IV dripped in, patients trickled in. Unlike previous days, there was little talking. I was engrossed in reading *The Traveler* in *Pictures in My Head* when I detected sobbing to my right.

A young man, about seventeen or eighteen years of age, cried as a nurse started his IV. Pale and gaunt in appearance, the baldheaded young man stared straight ahead. Tears ran down his cheeks. As the nurse hung a 250 ml IV bag, he turned to the woman beside him and said, "Please, Mom, make the pain stop."

The woman turned from him and cried.

A lump rose in my throat. I closed my eyes. Please, God, stop the suffering, I begged.

I experienced steady throbbing in my head and sinuses. I looked at my IV—only 100 ml left to go and I would be free. I had been cautioned to let the nurses know if I experienced sinus pressure, but I just wanted to get through the treatment, so I kept silent.

An elderly man shuffled in, carrying a portable oxygen tank. He sat down next to me. Patty hurried in, dragging a large oxygen tank behind her. She disconnected the man's tubing from the portable tank and hooked it up to the larger tank. Looking very weary, he leaned his head against the chair as she accessed his port. Deep furrows were etched across his forehead. He closed his eyes. His thin-skinned hands hung loosely over the arms of his chair, and a slight tremor became evident as he reached up to scratch his nose. He'd buttoned his dark brown sweater unevenly. It partially covered a tan shirt with a brown stain. His black pants hung loosely on him, cinched tightly with a cracked brown belt. He wore scuffed brown shoes without socks. His thinning patch of hair was uncombed. Senile lentigines—old age spots—covered his face. He coughed up phlegm and spit it into a Kleenex.

I closed my eyes. Would I have the courage to endure another round of chemotherapy? Some of the patients I met in the oncology office had experienced exacerbations of their cancer. Next time, the drugs would be more toxic, the side effects potentially horrendous, as they tried to destroy cells resistant to previous drugs.

I opened my eyes to Patty's hovering over me. My IV was finished. After pulling the catheter, Patty presented me with a coffee mug, emblazoned with a smiling stick figure leaping into the air with the single word, "Yippee!" inscribed upon it.

"Graduation present," she said, smiling.

"I've enjoyed meeting all the nursing staff, Patty. I hope I never see any of you in this treatment room again, although I wouldn't mind running into you in a bookstore."

I felt elated, free, exhilarated as I drove home. There would be no more Friday chemotherapy.

I made a quiche and salad for dinner, curled up with a blanket in front of the television and watched *The Brylcreem Boys*. I had become quite the movie connoisseur since my treatments began. Within an hour, nausea hit me and the pounding in my head became severe. I took two Tylenol and ate a piece of bread. My whole body ached with fatigue.

I fell asleep on the couch, only to wake to severe pounding in my head. The nausea worsened. I forced down a couple of ounces of ginger ale, and then shuffled to the bathroom—more urinary urgency. Looking in the mirror, my face had, for the sixth and final time, transformed into summer squash yellow—yellow had *never* been my color. Disgusted, I returned to the couch and covered my head with a blanket.

When Bill came home, he sat beside me and pulled the blanket off my head. "How are you feeling, Pam?"

"Emotionally I feel elated, but physically I feel like shit. Welcome home."

Sadness filled his eyes. He stroked my hair. The attention was nice. I wondered if gobs of hair would come out in his hand. Although my hair had thinned appreciably, there were no areas of baldness. I fooled people with hair spray, teasing what I had to give the illusion of volume. Maybe I just fooled myself.

After Bill and the kids polished off the quiche, he sat beside me, cradling my head in his lap—very nice. Heidi lay at my feet, her head covering my ankles. Bill and I watched *The Matchmaker*, the story of an American woman who stumbles upon a quaint Irish town's Matchmaking Festival while searching for her boss' Irish ancestors.

"I couldn't find the town *Baile Na Grá* anywhere in Ireland, Bill, but I did discover an annual Matchmaking Festival in the town of Lisdoonvarna in the West of Ireland. It's held during the month of September and the town swells from a population of under one thousand to over ten thousand. Maybe we could go someday," I suggested.

"Looking for a new husband?"

"No, I've decided to keep the one I have, thank-you very much."

Feeling worse, I went upstairs to lie down. I piled on blankets as I shivered uncontrollably. The shivering intensified the pounding in my head. I tossed and turned, unable to find a semi-comfortable position for my aching/shivering/nauseated/canary-colored body.

I woke up three times during the next couple of hours from the steady pressure in my head. I took ibuprofen but gained no relief. The next morning, I was up only an hour to start a load of laundry and eat a piece of toast before the pressure in my sinuses became unbearable and forced me to lie down. Over the course of the day, I stayed in bed, experiencing temperature extremes, during which I intermittently piled on and tossed off blankets. The sinus pain became so intense I vomited several times. Thankfully, I managed to hit the wastebasket. Every time I got up to use the bathroom— once or twice an hour—a sledgehammer pounded in my head and my fatigued limbs resisted movement.

Now I've got to add a comment here. Although I could blame much of my misery on the chemotherapy, I had no one but myself to blame for my intense sinus headache. I had been asked many times to alert the nursing staff to any sinus discomfort. They would have slowed down the drip. I'd been so stubborn during my last treatment, so intent on escaping, that I'd ignored that oft-repeated request. I'll just say: IT'S NOT WORTH IT!!

Instead of staying in the treatment area for an additional hour, I suffered for days. A word to the wise, as they say…

The next morning, I felt worse. I got up long enough to open a window. I took my mind off my miserable headache by concentrating on birds chirping and neighbors' children playing and arguing. It didn't help my headache, but it brought back memories of my own brood's youthful days. There's something satisfying in knowing other mothers suffer from sibling fights and rivalry. I smiled and rolled over, finally returning to sleep.

Later, Jon popped in to let me know he was whisking Rob off to CU to hang out with friends who'd recently rented a house off campus.

"Who rented the house?"

"Just my pals from the dorm: Kevin, Nick, Henri, Pat, and Jason."

"What's the house like?"

"It's awesome, Mom! It's perfect."

"Did they buy or rent furniture?"

"Furniture?"

"They don't have furniture?"

"Mom, it's a guys' house."

"Which means what, exactly?" The throbbing in my head intensified as I concentrated on the conversation.

"The guys threw a few mattresses on the floors. They've got hangers in the closet, an old pool table, a dartboard, seven-computer LAN, and a kegerator—all the necessities."

"Excuse my ignorance, but could you explain to your doddering fool of a mother what a LAN and kegerator are?"

"Sure. LAN is a local area network."

"That's clear as mud."

He didn't say anything for a minute. He was probably pondering the impossibility that such a computer-illiterate woman could possibly have given birth to him. "A LAN means the computers are all connected. It makes playing games and downloading files much faster."

"There must be a ton of cables."

"You should see it! It's awesome! It's like this huge rat maze running all over the place. And it keeps growing."

Ah, the things that excite the next generation. "And a kegerator?"

"Nick put a keg of beer in the refrigerator, got an automatic CO_2 tap, and drilled a hole through the door so you don't even have to open it to pour a beer."

"So there's only room for frozen foods."

"No. The freezer is where they store the hard liquor."

"Silly me. What else could they possibly need?"

"Not a thing."

"I was being facetious, Jon."

"Don't do that."

"It's a professional hazard. I was thinking like a mother. You know, beds, dressers, a few vegetables in the refrigerator..."

"Thinking like a mother can be painful, Mom. They do have a refrigerator for food, but the last time I looked in it, the only greens I saw were molds. There were a few hotdogs and fruit drinks to mix with the booze, but that's about it."

"Jon, as you like to say to me, 'that is definitely more information than I need'. Have a good time, but not too good a time. I think you know what I mean."

"I do. See you later."

"Don't forget Rob has a date tonight. He's taking Cheryl to the Broker Inn for dinner."

"I won't forget."

"I don't know if I have the stomach to ask this, Jon, but do you plan to eat lunch with your pals?"

"We'll grab some pizza." The pounding in my head increased. I moaned something and he shot out the door.

Heather stuck her head in to remind me she was going to the Air Force Academy to spend a couple days with her boyfriend. She hurriedly added she would spend the night at his sponsor's house so I wouldn't have to worry. I felt too sick to worry. Besides, if she thought I believed staying at a sponsor's house would prevent anything in particular, she was kidding herself. I wasn't born yesterday, although for some strange reason, the kids always thought Bill and I hadn't a clue about what they were up to. Considering I'd missed a few of their childhood escapades, maybe they weren't completely wrong.

"I'll be back tomorrow evening to help you celebrate Mother's Day," she promised.

"Don't worry about it. I don't believe this will be one of my happier Mother's Days, although it may be more memorable than others. Have a good time and drive safely. Please call when you get there."

It was night when I awoke to a gentle pressure at my side. Bill sat on the bed, holding my hand in the darkened room.

"Sorry you feel so miserable. I made out a grocery list and went to the store earlier. I even bought some broccoli, so you know I made an effort. I don't want you to worry about a thing. Just get better. Oh, Heather called to let us know she arrived in Colorado Springs safely."

I was touched. "Thank-you, Bill. I really, really appreciate it." I tried to move. "My legs are asleep."

"That's because I just shooed Hannah off the bed. She was sprawled across your lower legs."

He kissed me and I fell back asleep, waking later to the steady cacophony of his snoring. I walked downstairs. Heidi trotted beside me. Feeling less nauseated, I made myself some cocoa and ate half an apple. I decided to sleep in the guestroom rather than contend with Bill's log sawing.

...

I did not waken until 6:45 on Sunday morning. "Bill," I hollered up the stairs, "Mass starts in forty-five minutes. Can you get ready?" Hollering proved to be a serious mistake. The sinus pressure exacerbated.

"I'll go with you, Pam. After all, it's Mother's Day."

Within a few moments of arriving at church, I realized I'd made a serious mistake getting out of bed. Weakness and aching wracked my body. I grabbed Bill's sleeve.

"My God, you look pale all of a sudden," he commented quietly. "Are you all right?"

No, I wasn't all right, but I lied. "I'm fine. I just need to sit down."

He guided me to a pew and I sat for a couple of minutes, wishing the lightheadedness away before kneeling. I tried to concentrate on my prayers, but all I could think of was my desire to get back to bed. Wearily, I wished there were a cot tucked away in some alcove where I could stretch out. The sinus pressure escalated.

Seated, I glanced around at the renovations that had recently been completed. Increased seating accommodated the multiplying congregation. A vestibule had been added with a baptismal font large enough to immerse adults. The addition of a choir loft held extra seating and an organ.

Unlike many of the churches we'd belonged to during Bill's naval career, this was a *real* church, with stained glass windows. For the twenty years before we moved to Louisville, we'd contributed to several building funds and attended Masses in drafty auditoriums while the *real* churches were erected. Invariably, they were completed within a few months of Bill's receiving orders to a new base.

Home at last, Bill promised, "We'll celebrate Mother's Day next weekend. I'll take you to a nice brunch at the Broker Inn. Maybe there'll be a discount on all the leftovers from today's brunch."

Rob breezed into the bedroom. "Speaking of the Broker Inn," he grinned, "I have a funny story to tell you, Mom. Hopefully it will add a little something to your Mother's Day in spite of the fact you feel like dog do."

"And don't look any better than that, either," I interjected.

"I wouldn't have said that."

"I know, so I mentioned it for both of us. So, what hilarious anecdote do you wish to share with your humorously challenged mother today?"

He cleared his throat. "Last night I took Cheryl to the Broker Inn. As an appetizer, the waiter brought out a large bowl of boiled shrimp. Mom, since you're not fond of any shrimp that's not wrapped in batter, I don't remember ever having had boiled shrimp, but I figured I would give them a try. They seemed kind of crunchy, but I ate a couple. Cheryl looked at me kind of funny. Then she peeled a shrimp. Honest to God, I didn't know you had to peel them! Anyway, I tried to save face by telling her I grew up at the beach and people on the coast don't peel shrimp. Next thing I knew, she was eating one without peeling it. I felt kind of bad."

"I assume you told her the truth."

"The subject didn't come up again, so I guess I let her believe it."

"Please tell me you're joking."

"Nope."

"I'm going to have a chat with that young lady the next time I see her. I can't let her go through life thinking that beachcombers eat shrimp without peeling them. You're rotten, boy. However, that will have to wait. I plan to spend the day in bed, so I'll feel well enough to work tomorrow. You guys are on your own today. Have a nice Mother's Day without me."

"We'll try," Bill promised. "Actually, since I figured you wouldn't want us around anyway, Jon and I are playing golf. It wasn't hard getting a tee time, since most golfers are catering to their wives."

"Let's hope they are. You guys go ahead. Leave the dogs with me. I need to feel better by tomorrow."

...

Actually, I didn't make it to work on Monday or Tuesday. In fact, I barely made it through Wednesday and Thursday. I kept telling myself the worst was behind me. I would shortly be on the road to recovery.

Chapter 28 - June 4th

"Eilish, I need your help." I could hear a steady hum through the telephone, which indicated Rob was using the computer again. "Before I ask my favor, I want to thank you for all your phone calls over the past few months."

"Ah, you're very welcome, Pamalla. I know you're glad chemotherapy is over."

"I am indeed. Bill will be very happy when he doesn't have to work so hard around the house."

"You mean you're going to let him off the hook?"

"I won't have an excuse not to keep the house up any longer."

"And why would you need one? You tell Bill to keep up the good work. You deserve help."

"Thanks. I may just do that."

"What did you wish to ask me?"

"I'm trying to deny the radiation treatments coming up by planning a trip to Ireland."

"You're going for sure?"

"Bill promised. And I can always count on his promises. I have books on traveling in Ireland, moving to Ireland, Irish customs, history, and myths. I've maps galore, and tons of videos. I have so much material that I don't know where to begin. There's too much to pick from."

"It may seem a bit obvious, but you'll want to visit a few of the tourist traps during your first trip. Once you're there, it will be easier to find little out of the way places you'd like to visit. I would suggest you fly into Dublin and begin there. If you've a mind to see the language and cultural center of the country, you'll want to travel to Galway as well."

"How are the roads, Eilish?"

"In smaller towns, they're a bit of a challenge for sure. You'll be making more than a few Signs of the Cross as you pass within a hairsbreadth of oncoming cars. And there will surely be a few flocks of sheep or cows impeding your progress. Give yourself loads of time to get from one place to another if you're taking scenic routes. Major roads are much as they are in the States, although there are few such grand highways. You won't need a car in Dublin. Buses will take you anywhere you've a mind to go. If you find driving on small roads a challenge, you'll be taking your life in your hands in the capital city. However, once you head out of Dublin, a car would improve your chances of reaching your destinations before the close of the century."

"That's helpful advice, Eilish. Thanks."

"You've made comments about planning a novel in Ireland after you finish your book on breast cancer, Pamalla. Have you any particular county in mind as background for your book?"

"I do, as a matter of fact."

"Which one?"

"County Tipperary, Eilish."

"That's where I was born!"

"I know. That's why I picked it. I'm hoping you'll be kind enough to advise me so I don't get into trouble and make a *bollix* of everything. Would you consider that, Eilish?"

"I'd be happy to, but you know I left Ireland years ago."

"As will my heroine. Actually, I'm not ready to set the next book in Ireland, but I know enough to make my heroine an Irish emigrant. She'll experience nursing school as I did in the 1970s."

"So there's to be an autobiographical component to your book?"

"There will be. I've a few issues with those years to iron out. I've always read one should write what one knows."

"Have you chosen a name for your heroine?"

"I fancy Fiona. I'm not sure about the last name. How does O'Meara sound to you, Eilish?"

"Lovely! The O'Meara clan hails from the northern part of County Tipperary, if you didn't know that."

"I didn't, but thank-you, Eilish. This is great. You'll be a terrific help. I hope you really don't mind."

She chuckled. "I may live in the States now, but part of my heart remains in Ireland. I'll have no problem talking about my home there. I imagine you'll want to visit County Tipperary when you go to Ireland, Pamalla."

"I do. It's one of the places listed on my pilgrimage."

"A pilgrimage, is it?"

I laughed. "That probably sounds silly, but that's what I'm calling it. Since we'll be there only two weeks, I've narrowed it down to a few counties. Visiting Tipperary is near the top of the list. I want my novel to feel authentic."

"Good. I've an idea for an inexpensive place to stay, if that would suit you."

"I'm all ears, Eilish. The trip will be expensive, so any advice about saving money would be greatly appreciated."

"I've stayed at Mount St. Joseph's Abbey in Roscrea, Pamalla. The grounds are lovely and spending the night is quite reasonable. If you'd like, I'll find the number."

"Lovely. An abbey—what would you think of St. Joseph's as a setting for a murder? "

"Oh, you could plan a lovely murder there, Pamalla."

"The little wheels in my brain are turning."

"Are you thinking of changing your setting for your novel to Ireland itself now?"

"Oh goodness, no, Eilish. I'll need to do tons more research before I can set a novel in Ireland, even with my Irish-American characters. I'll need more than one visit to Ireland before I tackle that. I say that in hopes this will not be my only trip."

"You might not like Ireland when you get there, Pamalla."

"Fat chance! I'm excited about going, but I'm not going with any pre-conceived expectations, so I expect I'll have a lovely time."

"I hope you do."

"I'll need more Irish connections before I can plan a novel in Ireland," I said. "Maybe the second novel—I'm thinking of a lovely man, who works on the grounds of the abbey..."

"You're very ambitious, Pamalla."

"I'm a dreamer. I have two books to write and more research to do before I can begin such a novel. However, I know where I can find books on Tipperary."

"I don't think local bookstores have much in that department," she said.

"You're right, Eilish. The local selections are pitiful for my needs. But I've a friend who's put me onto a bookstore in County Galway that sends book parcels internationally. The owner will find available books for me."

"What's the name of the shop, Pam?"

"Kennys Bookshop in Galway City. I'm looking forward to visiting for a few hours when we're there. I'm told they've five floors of books."

"And will Bill enjoy that, do you think?"

"He loves bookstores too, but I think more than an hour will do him in. But hey, it's Ireland. Surely there'll be a pub or two in the vicinity where he can enjoy a couple of pints while he's waiting for me. We have to go to Kennys; it's on my pilgrimage list."

"It sounds like you've already given some thought to this pilgrimage list. What else is on it?"

I rummaged through my papers to find my list. Some day I'd have to get organized. "If we start out in Dublin, I want to visit the GPO—that's right isn't it, Eilish? People say GPO instead of the General Post Office?"

"That's right."

"Right. The GPO where Pádraic Pearse and his cohorts held off the English during the Easter Rising of 1916."

"Have you been studying the Easter Rising, Pamalla?"

"I have. Are you familiar with the book, *1916*, by Morgan Llywelyn, Eilish?"

"I'm not."

"It was actually the first book about Irish history I read. It's part novel and part non-fiction. Llywelyn chronicles the story of a young Irishman and his part in the Easter Rising. The courage of the leaders touched me deeply. They inspired my love of the Irish people. Despite hundreds of years of abuse, there were always the few who resisted oppression. It's like me fighting this cancer. I refuse to succumb without a fight."

"There's probably some psychological phenomenon to account for your passion."

"There probably is, but putting a name on it doesn't matter to me. I'm happy. You know what bothers me about the Easter Rising?"

"What, Pamalla?"

"The leaders died without knowing the people of Ireland would fight for freedom."

"By the time of the Rising, most Irish were tired of fighting, Pamalla. While Pearse and the others held strategic buildings in Dublin, citizens looted the city. They were desperately poor, disillusioned, and afraid of English reprisals. They pelted the rebel leaders with fruits and vegetables as they were marched to Kilmainham Gaol. However, the peoples' feelings changed when the leaders were murdered after trials that mocked justice."

"I read that. I want to visit Kilmainham Gaol, Eilish. It was used as a set in the movie, *In the Name of the Father*. That was an interesting tale—the story of the Guildford Four and the Maguire family. How could innocent people languish in prison for years despite absolute evidence proving their innocence?"

"It was a difficult time, with bombings in Northern Ireland and England. Arrests were made to appease frightened citizens. It was all terribly wrong—terribly. But people are striving to live together—to put the past behind them. Those who cause trouble in the North are a minority of citizens. Most people want peace."

"Those few seem to have loud voices, Eilish."

"They do. Are you planning a trip to the North?"

"Not this visit. I want to spend my time in the South, especially Galway and Dublin."

"What other stops have you put on your itinerary?" she asked.

"I want to visit the Dingle Peninsula."

"Ah, it's lovely. It really is. What draws you there?"

"I've read about the Great Blasket Islanders and their preservation of the Irish language and culture. I understand that if one stands at the tip of the peninsula in Dunquin, one can see the homes across the water that were abandoned on the Great Blasket Island in 1953."

"That depends on the weather. There's many a day it's too rainy and foggy to see a blessed thing."

"I'll pray for good weather."

"I'm not sure what advice about your trip you need from me, Pamalla. It sounds like you're doing fine planning the trip."

"But I have only the outline done. I need to fill in the gaps."

"If you're smart, you'll fill in the gaps once you get there. You don't want to pack in so much you forget to enjoy yourself. The Irish are a relaxed lot. Enjoy my people. Rest and recuperate. You've been through a great deal."

"Bill would like to rent a boat and travel down the Shannon River, stopping in at little towns along the way, but we'll have to leave that for another visit."

"A friend of mind did that nearly ten years ago, Pamalla. I expect things have changed a mite, but she told me everyone was quite friendly. There was always a pub or two where supplies could be had, like tins of meat, potatoes, bread, beer, and shrouds."

"Shrouds?"

"You never know when you might be needing one."

"Ah, the Irish. Always ready for anything."

"So it's been said. Speaking of which, if I don't get to the store, there'll be no supper for my husband tonight."

"Eilish, thanks for your help."

"You're welcome. Mind you don't plan too much, and you'll have a better time. Have a pleasant evening, Pamalla."

Chapter 29 - June 14th

With a sense of foreboding, I pulled into the parking lot of the Miriam R. Hart Regional Radiation Therapy Center in Boulder. I took a deep breath before turning off the ignition and returning both hands to the wheel. My fingers gripped it so tightly they throbbed. Unwilling to move, I stared straight ahead at the brick, one-story building that would be a daily reminder of my cancer for the next five weeks. I exhaled forcefully.

With chemotherapy behind me, and my fatigue waning ever so slightly, I'd clothed myself in denial to regain a modicum of normalcy and the teeniest bit of control over my life. Physically, radiation should have fewer side effects, but emotionally, I was a basket case, the stark reality of another treatment regimen looming before me.

Leaden-footed, I walked over to the receptionist's desk. A middle-aged woman flashed a wide grin. "Good morning. How may I help you?"

I tried to return the smile despite the trepidation I felt; it felt forced and unnatural. After introducing myself, I was directed to a row of padded chairs to wait while the receptionist gathered papers for my chart. Biding my time, I studied an imposing quilt that hung on the opposite wall, a brilliant patchwork of greens, pinks, and purples. The hand-sewn work of art included brightly colored humming birds flitting about a cluster of irises, cattails, lilies, and a few flowers that represented the poetic license of a creative mind. The quilt accented the room, which was decorated in subtle shades of purple and aqua. It put Dr. Sitarik's office in mind. I wondered if there was a central clearinghouse for decorators of oncology waiting rooms, with a lone figure determining that "shades of mauves and greens are least disruptive to the damaged psyche of the terminally ill".

A coffee machine beckoned at one end of the sitting room, cups and non-dairy creamer at the ready. Okay, it didn't beckon to me; I never developed a taste for coffee and couldn't choke down a cup if my life depended on it. I read about some study asking Americans if they'd give up their daily cup of coffee for $1000 a week. A resounding majority said, "No!" They didn't ask me. I'd gladly avoid coffee for the rest of my life for a grand a week—or a month, for that matter.

Three corridors branched off the waiting area to parts unknown. I fidgeted in my chair. Uncharacteristically, I chewed my fingernails. Nervousness pummeled me. After an interminably long few minutes, I was led to a small room. Sitting at a desk half-facing me, the receptionist, whose name escaped me the moment I heard it, said, "Darn insurance forms—I'll ask you the questions and fill in the paperwork. Then the doctor will see you."

Forms completed, I was escorted to a small cubicle where I exchanged my clothes for a stylish blue, goose-bump-producing thin cotton gown with *Boulder Community Hospital* printed in black lettering across the front. I harbored a suspicion that the hardly subtle block lettering would not deter hardened kleptomaniacs, but I suspected few women would be caught dead in such a drape if given an alternative—forgive the unfortunate choice of words. I had to admit, however, that having seen clips from recent haute couture fashion shows, there might be a market for hospital gowns stamped with various slogans and catch phrases. After all, there were at least two basic styles—the more popular open-backed and breezily sensuous gown, as well as the three-arm-hole "which way does this *fecking* thing go on" wrap-around model. With a multitude of colors and prints and a bit of imagination—perhaps a tassel here and some fringe there—Vera Wang or Bob Mackie might beg for the opportunity to develop such a line. Supermodels would be perfect to encourage sales. Surely the pinched, emotionless expressions I'd seen on the emaciated faces of most models trotting down runways were more doleful than any sallow, pained expression I'd displayed during the worst of my chemo—including puking in the trash can.

I placed my belongings in a locker and reflected that several hundred fewer calories wouldn't hurt me now and again. Soberly, I walked to an examination room across the hall. The exam room was large enough to summersault across. It was easily double, perhaps triple, the size of the largest such room at the Family Medical Center.

Imagine being able to examine a patient without being wedged between the table and sink! There was no evidence of rain-stained ceiling panels or peeling wallpaper. No cupboards stood partially open because of warped cabinet doors. The air smelled fresh, unlike in our clinic, where a rat had crawled into a heating vent, died, and practically asphyxiated staff and patients.

"God, we need a new place!" I muttered aloud, though no one was within hearing distance of my heartfelt remark. I shivered; there was nothing wrong with the air conditioning in the radiation oncology building either. Goose bumps crept over my arms and legs.

The door opened and a good-looking man entered. He wore a white lab coat over a tan silk shirt and dark brown pants. His tie sported an assortment of fly-fishing lures and paraphernalia. Extending his hand, he pumped mine and introduced himself as Dr. McNeely, the radiation oncologist.

"I've read your surgical and chemotherapy reports, Mrs. Stockho. Except for pharmacology, this will be the final phase of your treatment. I assume Dr. Sitarik has discussed your taking tamoxifen after radiation treatments have been completed?"

"He has. I'll start the medication later this summer."

"Excellent. For the next few minutes, I would like to explain what to expect from us. I have tried to anticipate the most common questions, but feel free to verbalize any concerns as we proceed. After I complete an examination, Debbie, one of our radiation therapists, will assist me in mapping out the area of radiation treatment. Our goal is to cover the area affected by cancer while minimizing exposure of healthy underlying tissues, like your lungs and heart. Very precise measurements will be entered into our computer. Many people, doctors included, figure that all we radiation oncologists do is aim and shoot. It's much more complicated than that.

"We direct X-ray beams at the affected area tangentially, that is, angled both downwards and upwards at the breast. Over the next couple of days, we will create a unique mathematical model, based on our measurements today, which will determine exact angles to direct your X-ray beams. Some of the variables that will enter into this computer-based model include the contours of your breast and ribcage, as well as the location of the tumor. The measurements we take today and the mathematical model developed from those measurements will be relayed to the treatment computer. Every time you are positioned for treatment, the radiation beam will be aimed in the same place. We allow enough of a margin to accommodate slight daily variations in positioning, breathing, minor weight changes, and breast swelling. The daily dose is exactly the same. Any questions so far?"

"It sounds complicated."

"That's how we earn our money," Dr. McNeely laughed. "After I examine you, Debbie will escort you to another room and take measurements. She will use a magic marker to reflect the measured area and take Polaroid pictures that will be added to your permanent chart. You will receive several tiny, permanent tattoos on your breast. The therapist will match them up with laser cross hairs to ensure that the same area is treated each time. There are three separate laser cross hairs used for alignment to ensure precision: two are emitted from opposite walls and the third is emitted from the ceiling. They meet centrally. The treatment machine illuminates the area to be irradiated. Debbie will also take X-rays today that will show the proposed area of treatment, so we can correctly position the Gantry arm, which is the moveable piece of the radiation machine."

I looked at him blankly. I was no idiot, but he was throwing a lot of information at me, and I thought I was picking up maybe every second or third word. I wondered how many patients really understood what they were being told. I didn't want to do this; I'd had enough already. But the clinical practitioner took over, reminding me that chemo and radiation were hedging my bets against recurrence and death.

Like others contemplating cancer treatment, I'd wanted to dismiss invasive treatments that made me feel so miserable, but I never felt comfortable putting my trust in isolated anecdotal accounts. Although I wanted to yell, "Hooray!" for cancer-free individuals who injected plant derivatives into their thighs every day or chewed exotic fruit pits, I felt security in numbers—big ones—that showed remission of cancer for thousands, hundreds of thousands, even millions who exposed themselves to treatments now being proposed for me. In my heart, I knew I might be one of the failures, but there was comfort in big numbers. Soon, research would lead us down entirely new paths to treat cancer, including the ability to genetically determine which cancers were more likely to metastasize, thereby sparing some women chemotherapy; I prayed it would be soon. But right now...

Having said that, I also had to admit I was frequently as frustrated as everyone else who followed recommendations outlined in verifiable research that was contradicted by equally verifiable research a few years later. I often threw up my hands and screamed, "What do I tell patients?"

Although patients hope medical practitioners have the answers for all baffling health questions, medicine is a constantly developing science. We can only work with information we have. I try to keep up with current research to reassure patients I take their health concerns as seriously as if they were my own. I encourage patients to actively participate in their care by researching treatments for their medical problems. I do warn them that not everything listed on the Internet is true, but we review material together and decide on a plan of action that is acceptable to both them and me.

I am always thrilled to meet a practitioner of Western medicine who has the foresight to incorporate other healing arts into his or her practice, like acupuncture or Chinese herbs. However, it worries me that unlike many countries, we do not regulate over-the-counter herbs. Many Americans choose herbal preparations without understanding their mechanisms of action, which may affect other medications, create surgical risks, and impact negatively on existing health problems. And that's not even considering the lack of standardization from pill to pill and bottle to bottle. I always ask my patients about over-the-counter herbal preparations they use. That arms me with knowledge to advise them about potential interactions and risks. I encourage patients to seek the advice of licensed herbalists who understand drug/herb interactions and can provide standardized herbal preparations.

I wholeheartedly supported maximizing my chances for survival by incorporating alternative treatments into my health plan, including fine-tuning my attitude through prayer when I wasn't bawling my eyes out. I'd thrown stress-lessening biofeedback into my *strive for health* milkshake. I'd added more fruits, vegetables, and whole grains to my diet. I had toyed with the idea of incorporating acupuncture and acupressure to help with nausea and pain.

I glanced at Dr. McNeely and wondered if he thought my silence an affirmation of my understanding, or did he realize I was in shock, numb from recent cancer treatments and reticent about undertaking more physical abuse.

"Do you have any questions so far, Pam?"

I shook my head and murmured, "No, sir."

"Fine. Now that the mechanical explanation is out of the way, I'd like to talk about possible physical effects. It is very common to experience some redness, like sunburn, over the entire breast and axilla. We treat the entire breast, Pam, not just the area where cancer was removed, because cancer cells may have migrated to other areas of the breast. Studies are underway to determine if there is a statistically significant difference in irradiating the entire breast as opposed to just the quadrant containing the cancer, but results have not yet been published."

His statement hit me hard and unexpectedly. I could be considered a statistic, a number, a decimal point, a percentage—one of those individuals who rounded out studies that I so blatantly defended as important when considering therapeutic options. Those women were just as real as I, just as scared, and just as hopeful. Their lives were every bit as important as my own. Many lived and many died.

My chest felt heavy, and I fought back tears. My sudden ability to go from exhilaration to despair still constantly amazed me. I wondered if I should talk to Gloria Bachelder about starting an anti-depressant, although that answer didn't seem right either. Feeling depressed about my current state of health had to be normal. God knew cancer wasn't a romp through a wildflower-filled park. I was daydreaming again instead of listening to my doctor. Maybe catching just the odd word was my poor attempt to cope.

"Breast redness may increase for up to a month after treatments end, as damaged cells continue to die and the healing process begins. The radiation does not remain in the breast. Some women are more sensitive to these breast changes than others. For women who burn rather than tan, for instance, we may lower the dose per treatment and increase the total number of treatments. The cumulative dosage is the same. Over five weeks, you will receive five thousand rads. You may also experience discomfort or pain in the breast, especially in the area where the mass was removed. That is normal. When we check your progress weekly, we'll ask you to apprise us of side effects. Debbie will discuss breast care while she takes measurements today."

After he checked my breasts and axillae, he further examined the area where the tumor had been excised, now only palpably noticeable by the one-centimeter, slight depression that remained above the red incision line. Dr. McNeely noted I had what some providers call fibrocystic tissue—lumpy boobs. It's actually a normal type of breast tissue.

"People call this type of tissue fibrocystic, but I prefer to think of it as cobblestones," he said.

Once the exam ended and talking about radiation therapy was over, my mood improved. "I have a joke for you since you brought up the subject of cobblestones, Dr. McNeely." I eased my arms back into my gown. I always felt better when I could remember a joke. "It seems two nuns were riding their bicycles through town on their way back to the convent after working in the local soup kitchen. Sister Mary Patrick says to her companion, 'Sister, would you mind if we take another route to the convent? We're always going back the same way.' 'Of course,' her companion assures her, whereupon she heads down a back street. After a couple of minutes, Sister Mary Patrick says, 'I've never *come* this way,' to which her companion replies, 'It's the cobblestones, Sister.' " I waited as the doctor absorbed the joke and laughed. Reaction to that punch line usually took a moment or two.

"You might share that joke with Debbie, Pam. She appreciates a good laugh."

As Debbie walked me down the hall to the mapping room, I admired a number of exquisite pencil drawings of children and dogs. "These are wonderful, Debbie."

"They were given to us by a patient, Pam. Her case was tragic. She was a woman in her thirties who belonged to a religious group that did not believe in medical intervention of any kind. Her husband refused to let her seek treatment, even though she found the breast lump when it was very small. She wanted treatment so her four small children could grow up with a mother. She finally left her husband, moved here with the kids, changed her name, and sought medical help. Unfortunately, by that time, the breast cancer had metastasized to the bone. We did what we could. She lived for five years after treatment—five years she might not have had without medical intervention."

"That's so sad. She was truly gifted."

Debbie stopped and turned to me. "Pam, I'm sorry. There is so much loss around here we don't always think. I don't want to depress you."

"Oh, that's all right. I'm a nurse. Death is always difficult, but to lose a young mother is distressing."

"It is, especially when the outcome of her cancer might have been different had she sought help earlier."

"What happened to her children?"

"They were adopted by a wonderful family. Of course, it doesn't make up for the loss of their mother, but at least they're happy. I don't understand people who refuse medical intervention."

"I have a hard time with that, too, Debbie, but faith is a powerful motivator of behavior." Debbie's caring behavior lightened the sadness that I felt.

We arrived at another cold room, with an equally cold metal table. A large machine, with what I assumed to be a Gantry arm, was positioned over the table.

"This will probably feel a bit uncomfortable." Debbie grabbed a stepstool to help me onto the table. The unyielding cold metal table bit into my back. Debbie eased a pillow under my knees, relieving the pressure in my lower back. She helped me remove my arm from my gown, exposing the left side of my chest. Debbie placed my left arm in armrests that pulled it outward and back from the rest of my body. Guided by temporary marks placed on my breast by Dr. McNeely, which mapped out the treatment volume, Debbie began (what seemed like) the interminably long process of taking precise measurements. In truth it was a mere fifty minutes, but lying on a hard cold surface, with my breast exposed and my arm held away from my body, I would have sworn hours passed. I shivered as Debbie made frequent treks down the hall to Dr. McNeely's office. Goose bumps formed over every square inch of body surface.

My discomfort increased. Miserably, I wished for a warm blanket. I tried to trick my mind by picturing myself lying on a sandy beach, listening to waves lapping the shore. It didn't work. The closest I could come to approximate the cold I felt was lying on the beach while a hurricane swept the shores of Connecticut in the dead of winter. I was afraid to move, lest that disturb any of the work Debbie had diligently completed. I suppose I could have asked for a blanket, but that would have taken a wee bit of common sense. Of course poor Debbie couldn't read my mind, could she? I hate making a pest of myself, although complaining in a book doesn't seem to bother me too much.

Debbie returned from another jaunt down the hall. "Dr. McNeely is very pleased with the measurements. He and another radiation oncologist, Dr. Aarestad, concur. I'm going to take a couple of X-ray pictures, so Dr. McNeely can check the treatment volume. X-rays show the breast tissue and underlying structures."

Unable to speak without my teeth chattering, I merely nodded. In just a few moments, though, the X-rays were completed and Debbie scurried off, films in hand.

When she returned, she was beaming. "With your rounded ribcage and the high location of your tumor, Dr. McNeely was afraid it might be difficult to direct the beams without damage to surrounding tissue, but it won't be a problem. Tomorrow, we'll construct lead blocks to protect tissues we don't want to irradiate. They will be installed in the treatment machine before each session. We're nearly done, Pam. I only need to place permanent tattoos on your breast and take some Polaroid pictures."

"You won't be sending those Polaroids to any skin magazines will you?" I joked. "I wouldn't want to scare anyone expecting to see young, firm breasts."

"These will be put in your patient file. Only the doctors will look at them."

"I knew there was something kinky about radiation oncologists, Debbie. There is something definitely strange about people who keep pictures of breasts decorated with purple magic marker. When will my treatments begin? My insurance company approved today's planning session, but they indicated the treatment plan and subsequent referral would come from you."

Debbie stopped writing in my chart and walked to my side. She helped peel my back from the metal table. I sat up and tucked my breast into my gown.

"For this type of cancer, the standard of care is twenty-five radiation treatments. You'll come here Monday through Friday for five weeks. We've never had insurance company delays for standard cancer treatment. How about starting treatments this Thursday morning?"

"That would be fine. Any chance of an early morning appointment so I won't inconvenience our clinic too much?"

"How about eight-fifteen? Although today's session was a little long, once you return for treatments, you'll be in and out within ten to fifteen minutes. We'll direct X-ray beams at your breast from opposite angles, each one on for about forty-five to fifty seconds. We program a specific number of rads into the machine rather than a specific time period, so the exact number of seconds may vary a bit."

"Eight-fifteen sounds fine. I should be at work and ready to see patients by nine o'clock every day. Thanks, I appreciate it."

"Oh, a couple more things, Pam. You should know that one of the doctors will want to see you each Monday right after your radiation treatment. He will examine you, check your progress, and ask about side effects. Most women have some redness of the entire breast and some irritation of the nipple and those areas that tend to hold moisture, like the axilla and the skin under your breast. Keep those areas dry. Cornstarch is useful. Treat irritated skin with a moisturizer, like aloe gel, which we can give you here. Some ladies use vitamin E oil instead. Avoid lotions that contain scents, because they may irritate your skin. An absorbent cloth, like a handkerchief, is a practical solution to moisture. Airing out your breast by removing your bra in the evening may also decrease irritation and moisture. As the treatments progress, you may experience pain around the treated area. Start caring for your breast before you have symptoms to help decrease the possibility of side effects. If you have any problems either during or after your treatments, please call us. Additional therapies and pain medications are available. Hopefully, that's about it. Any questions?"

I shook my head. Debbie helped me off the table and showed me back to the dressing room where I changed and headed out of the building. I had thirty minutes to get back to the office before my afternoon appointments began. I was glad that kind people like Debbie would be helping me through my treatments!

Chapter 30 - June 17th

In spite of my hope I'd be seeing Debbie again, I wasn't terribly excited when I arrived for my first radiation treatment. The receptionist escorted me to the treatment waiting area after I changed into another lovely thin, blue gown. She gestured me toward a couch.

"The radiation therapist will look for you here each morning," she said pleasantly and walked away.

Seated on the couch beside me was a gray-haired, angelic-looking, cheerful woman of about seventy-five. Believe me, she didn't look that old, but when I told her I was writing the book, she insisted I put in her actual age.

"Hi!" she beamed. "I'm Nadine, from Estes Park. This is my seventh radiation treatment; eighteen to go and I'm out of here."

"My name's Pam. This is my first treatment, and I'm a bit nervous. Do you drive down from Estes Park every day?" Estes Park is at least a forty-five minute drive from Boulder.

"Every day. The ride's not too bad most days and the scenery is glorious. I give myself an extra fifteen minutes in case traffic is a bear. I don't want to be late for my appointment. At least these treatments provide proof my cancer's being given a run for the money, Pam. Do you have breast cancer, too?"

"I do, Nadine. I didn't have to suffer a mastectomy though—just a lumpectomy."

"Me, too," she said. "I guess there are different treatments based on how much surgery you have."

"As well as the type of breast cancer and one's age," I added.

"You certainly don't look old enough to be retired, Pam. Do you work?"

"I'm a nurse practitioner in family practice."

"One of my nieces is finishing her nurse practitioner training. She'll receive her master's degree in August. Do you enjoy what you do?"

"I love it. It would be even better to practice in a building as nice as this one. It must make everyone happy to come to work, which is probably a good thing considering the clientele."

"Do you see a lot of patients with cancer where you work, Pam?"

"More than I'd like, but since cancer treatments are constantly improving, many of us live long, productive lives. I remember taking care of women who had breast cancer surgery when I was in nursing school. There were no choices. The whole breast was lopped off, including muscle tissue underneath. All lymph nodes were removed from under the arm. A woman was often left with an ugly scar, decreased ability to move her arm, and permanent swelling along her entire arm. Talk about self-esteem issues! Now, at least, there are choices as well as reconstruction options. Even though some women still suffer permanent arm swelling within the first five to ten years after surgery, lymphedema specialists provide preventive counseling and physical therapy when needed. I'm not thrilled to have cancer, but at least I don't feel like a violated piece of meat."

"You sound passionate, Pam."

"I've been told that many times, Nadine. I take patients' rights seriously. A person needs to understand options to make informed decisions about treatments. Besides, having patients participate in planning their care takes some pressure off me."

"Nadine, we're ready for you," Debbie, our lovely radiation therapist, called from the hallway. I moved a little to one side to avoid attack by an overgrown potted philodendron that cascaded from a shelf hanging over the couch.

"I'll see you tomorrow, Pam. It's been nice meeting you. I hope my niece will feel as strongly about patient rights as you do."

"Nice to meet you, too, Nadine. Keep your spirits up."

Within five minutes, a beaming Nadine returned. "Next. There's nothing to it. It's a breeze."

"I'm glad to hear it." I rose to follow Debbie. "I'll see you tomorrow, Nadine."

Debbie led me down a corridor to another cold, metal table with an imposing X-ray machine looming overhead. As she helped me position my head and left arm, I studied a beautifully painted mural on the ceiling. Scores of green leaves flanked the majestic Flatirons. A galaxy of stars illuminated a dark blue sky.

"Barbara Fisher, a local artist, painted the mural, Pam. If you look carefully, you can pick out heads of people that have been creatively concealed among the leaves. She also hid several animal heads among the Flatirons."

As the Gantry arm was positioned to my left, I scrutinized the mural, finding a number of smiling faces hidden among the leaves, as well as a Buffalo head sculpted within the beautiful Flatirons. Over the next few days, additional hidden heads revealed themselves.

"The mural's absolutely magnificent," I remarked as my protective lead shields were placed in the machine. The entire wall to my right was divided into cubbyholes, each holding differently shaped lead shields, and each inscribed with a patient's name. While I focused on the cubbyholes, the laser cross hairs were aligned with the tattoos on my breast.

"Pam, you'll hear a humming noise as the beam turns on. I'll be back after the treatment is over. We'll take an X-ray of both treatment angles today for Dr. McNeely to review. After today, we'll take X-rays once a week. This ensures him our radiation technique is precise."

"I appreciate precision," I whispered.

"Just one more comment before I leave. These machines are designed to irradiate only a very specific area. Unlike X-rays found at the low end of the voltage spectrum, like those used for dental and chest X-rays, where the radiation is diffusely scattered, these X-rays are found at the high end of the spectrum, where they are more concentrated, with little scattering. You do not have to worry about your ovaries receiving radiation. A lead apron like those used when you have a chest X-ray is unnecessary. Some patients insist on wearing a lead apron, and we are happy to accommodate them, but I promise that no part of your body, other than your breast, is receiving any radiation. Do you feel comfortable with that?"

"Yes, Debbie." I appreciated her concern. "I know the thought behind radiation is to destroy remaining cancer cells, but doesn't it damage healthy cells as well? Can't cancer develop from those damaged, previously healthy cells?"

"You're right, Pam. Healthy cells are damaged as well. They usually either die or repair themselves. That's one of the big differences between healthy and cancerous cells. Healthy cells are much more capable of repair. Cancer cells are very simple cells."

"Why are there so many treatments, Debbie?"

"Cells are much more likely to die if hit by radiation during their mitotic, or dividing phase, Pam. We want to attack as many cancer cells as possible while they're dividing, and multiple treatments give us a better chance of doing that. Also, lower doses of radiation are given over time, rather than all at once, to significantly lessen the side effects. The incidence of cancer caused by this type of radiation is extremely small."

Debbie left the room and closed the door. She sat at a monitoring station with three computers and a video camera that assured her I did not move or sneeze during my treatment. The multiple computers provided safeguards for me; they verified that the radiation dosage and mathematical parameters determined for me were set correctly. Thinking about that made me think of myself as an algebraic equation. Chemo, radiation, and drug treatments on one side equaled a cancer cure on the other. Yeah! I could live with that.

Debbie scanned the monitors as a humming sound began and continued for about forty-five seconds. I understood there was a big difference between being exposed to a single dose of 5,000 rads and being exposed to a cumulative 5,000 rad dose over a series of treatments. My risk of complications was significantly decreased with low, daily doses. I stared at the Flatirons mural as the X-ray beams did their work.

•••

I looked forward to seeing Nadine. She was a gifted artist, an expert in still life paintings, and had been recognized as a master painter by the National Society of Tole and Decorative Painters. For years, she taught art classes, encouraging students to open their eyes to their surroundings.

"Many of us go through life with blinders on," she mused one day. "People seem so intent on earning money. They forget to stop and smell the roses, if you'll forgive my purloining that over-used expression. It's as if people go through life with blurred vision, unable to focus on the beauty around them. Do you know what I mean?"

"I do, Nadine, and I plead guilty. I can't say I've had a huge personality change since I found this cancer—and some would claim I've become a bit manic-depressive—but I'm enjoying life more. Sometimes I look out a window and experience life in the same wondrous way I did as a child. I've been fascinated watching a robin. She built a nest in one of the hanging baskets outside my kitchen window. Besides bits of straw, she's used pieces of dog hair to soften the nest. There are three blue eggs in the nest. I love watching her sit on those eggs. I'm eagerly awaiting the day when there will be three chirping babies. I don't think I've been so excited about birds in quite a while. I admire people who maintain that child-like awe throughout their lives. They don't need to be hit over the head with a two-by-four to appreciate life. Gosh, I'm sounding a bit maudlin today. Sorry."

"That's okay, Pam. I feel that way about Estes Park all the time. I relish its beauty each day. One sometimes forgets there are real problems outside our little valley community."

"It must be so gratifying to express yourself creatively through your painting, Nadine. I'd love to see your work. How about if I drive up to Estes Park and take you out to lunch after my treatments are completed, since you'll finish first?"

"That sounds great, but we'll go Dutch. We've all got to watch our pennies."

"How long did you teach painting?"

"For over thirty years. I loved it. It's so important to encourage students. I always tried to say at least one nice thing about a student's work, even if it was complimenting the way a single leaf was drawn on a tree. Years ago, a student told me I had pretty eyes. Do you understand what she meant?"

"I'm not sure."

"She meant I tried to see something positive and beautiful no matter how much effort it took. And I still do; it's a point of pride for me. Although it was very difficult to see anything positive about the incident that happened yesterday, believe me."

"What happened?"

"I spilled a bottle of India ink," Nadine said. "The cap had not been screwed on tightly. Now my beige carpet has a large, unsightly purple stain. I made it worse by rubbing the area. The cleaners are coming tomorrow, but I have a sinking feeling we'll have to replace the whole thing. What a mess. I couldn't think of anything positive about that."

"It would be difficult to find anything positive about replacing a carpet, Nadine."

"It'll be fine. Maybe the cleaners will have some luck removing the stain."

"I don't know about you, Nadine, but I see a scrub-clad therapist gesturing madly at one of us. It must be time for treatments again. They're always interrupting our conversations."

Nadine laughed. "We'll have to make up for all these short conversations when you come to Estes Park. While I'm gone, you might enjoy looking at some photographs I brought. My husband and I love riding his motorcycle. I also included pictures of still life paintings I've done."

"Wow!" I said, studying the pictures as she walked down the hall. "You look great in clothes. These blue gowns just don't do you justice." Nadine chuckled as she turned the corner.

...

Within a few short weeks, I bid Nadine and the wonderful radiation staff adieu. Nadine and I had bonded easily, and I doubted it was merely because we shared the same diagnosis. No, I was convinced Nadine was a gift from God, an angel in disguise, placed on earth to bring joy to those she encountered on life's journey. On her last day, Nadine presented tiny, framed pictures of exquisitely painted roses and peaches to the radiation therapists and me. I will treasure my paintings forever, for they remind me of one of the dearest angels who ever graced the earth.

Chapter 31 - August 6th

Nearly a month had passed since my last radiation treatment. My heart was lighter than when I'd last darkened the doorway of Dr. Sitarik's office. Gone were the bouts of nausea and vomiting. Most of the stabbing breast pains had been replaced by persistent axillary burning and aching under my arm, but even those discomforts were waning. The rashes were fading. I felt renewed and thankful and hopeful.

"Tell me how you're feeling, Pam," Dr. Sitarik encouraged.

"Almost like my old self."

"Did you have any problems with radiation?"

"I did. There was a bit of redness and discomfort during treatments, but that wasn't bad. However, three days after my treatments ended, discomfort escalated to excruciating pain. I couldn't sleep."

"Did you take anything for pain?"

"Ibuprofen didn't touch it. I don't like narcotics, but by the fourth night, I was so sleep deprived I took a hydrocodone, and it helped. I knew side effects of radiation could continue for up to four weeks after completion of treatments, but I didn't expect so much pain. I expected my underarm would be more affected than my breast because of the difference in tissue density. Of course, it probably didn't help that the tumor was so high in my breast."

"You had more reaction to the radiation than other patients I've had. Didn't the radiation oncology office offer anything to soothe it?"

"They did. They provided an aloe gel and two types of cream. But they didn't touch the pain."

"You should have called the clinic. They might have had additional treatments to ease your pain."

"You're right, doc. I should have called. Debbie mentioned something about gel pads for severe pain. I didn't remember about it at the time. Interestingly, my friend, Nadine, who is almost thirty years older than I, had practically no pain or tissue sloughing from her radiation treatments, and they were the same as mine. Now my only complaint is the numb feeling that's persisted along the back of my arm. It's maddening at times. Sometimes, I get an itchy feeling, but when I scratch the area, it just aches with numbness. The itch isn't satisfied. Does that sound weird?"

"No, it's not uncommon and may persist for several months to years."

"I sure like to complain, don't I?"

"I asked if you had any problems, as I recall."

"And I dumped them all on you. So, doc, what's the plan?"

"After I examine you, we'll discuss tamoxifen to decrease your risk of breast cancer recurrence. Slip on this gown and I'll be back shortly."

A couple of minutes later, he looked at my breasts, commenting that the amount of burn and peeling was about what he expected. After I lay down, he palpated both breasts and axillae, checked my lymph nodes, lungs, heart, and abdomen. He pronounced me in great shape, metaphorically speaking.

After I dressed, he sat in a chair in front of me. "Are you ready to start tamoxifen?"

"I'm not sure. I know it's the right thing to do, but I'm not crazy about the idea."

"Do you have any questions?"

"I don't think so. I know it blocks estrogen in the breast, but acts like estrogen in other tissues, like the uterus, bones, and liver. It may help prevent osteoporosis and decrease bad cholesterol."

"But..." he started.

"But? Oh, you mean there's an increased risk of endometrial cancer."

"Right. But the increase is small and that uterine problem has been found mainly in post-menopausal women."

"I promise if I take the drug, I will get annual exams and watch for weird periods. Of course, since chemo and tamoxifen will probably keep me menopausal, I'm not sure how I'm going to tell if there are endometrial problems."

"Just keep your doctor informed of any changes in your health or periods. Okay?"

"I will."

"Pam, you said, 'if I take the drug'. If?"

"Look, Doctor Sitarik, I'm not too crazy about putting more stuff in my body right now. I'm not thrilled about the potential for side effects, like going through menopause early. Granted, I haven't had a period since before my fourth treatment, which I don't mind at all, but I don't relish the idea of sitting down with a patient and sweating all over her after turning beet red from a hot flash."

"That may not happen, Pam."

"Right. And pigs may fly, too. My eyes are bad enough without the potential for this drug influencing them. I don't want to end up on anti-depressants because tamoxifen may cause depression. I've worked hard to keep my weight down and I'm not interested in bloating. I am not thrilled about the small, but real, possibility of blood clots. I feel pretty good right now and don't want to rock the boat."

"This medication may prevent a recurrence of your cancer, Pam."

"I know. And you probably think I'm nuts even questioning taking every avenue available to me to prevent its return."

"You're not nuts. Maybe a little scared."

"Maybe a lot scared."

"Pam, you know it's the responsibility of drug companies to advise patients of all potential side effects. Most women tolerate tamoxifen very well and experience little, if any, problem. How many drugs do you pre-scribe on a daily basis? There isn't a medication available that doesn't have a host of side effects listed in the PDR. You never see most of them in the general patient population. The bottom line is that, at this time, tamoxifen is your best chance to prevent a recurrence of breast cancer. Other preventive measures may be available in the next few years, but research hasn't been completed. I'm going to write the prescription for tamoxifen. You give it some thought. If you start it, I'd like to see you in about a month. If you do not start it, please call me."

"In other words, you want me to take it."

"I do."

"I'll think about it, Dr. Sitarik."

"That's all I ask for now."

...

Before I left the clinic, I stopped in to see the treatment nurses. Those six chemotherapy sessions were still very much in mind. A chill shot through me and I shook momentarily. I don't know what I'd expected— maybe that the color in the room would have changed or maybe I'd feel differently now that it was over. But that old feeling of apprehension stuck to me like a heavy overcoat on a humid day.

Today, only three people sat in green loungers. I wondered if I'd appeared to the nurses like these people did to me: frightened, sad, pale, and, and lost. One gentleman caught my attention. He was thin, jaundiced, and appeared despondent. An Avalanche ball cap covered his bald head. He looked up, fixed his gaze on me and smiled. His eyes sparkled. In that moment, I recognized him, but I couldn't believe how much he'd changed. It was Stan Lieberman, my patient with testicular cancer.

I'd talked to the Liebermans often and Sheila kept me abreast of Stan's condition. She cried often. Her young husband had endured five hospitalizations since his back surgery. He'd recovered some use of his legs after the spinal mass was removed. His slow, unsteady, hunched-over gait reminded her of a wizened old man. He could not move without the support of his walker. His bladder control returned and they were grateful, but he'd suffered horrendous complications from his chemotherapy.

He'd been home less than a week after his back surgery when Sheila rushed him to the hospital with severe chest pain and difficulty breathing. He'd suffered multiple pulmonary emboli—blood clots in his lungs that could have killed him at any moment. After he was heparinized (given medication to help dissolve clots and prevent formation of others), he returned home on oral blood thinners. His precarious medical condition, however, had contributed to difficulty regulating his clotting time. Sheila rushed him to the hospital once more when his gums and nose bled profusely. He urinated bright red blood. He remained in the hospital for several days while his medication levels were adjusted. His blood counts remained low. Not only was he anemic, but he also lacked any ability to combat germs breathed and coughed on him. Death lingered near his door.

Indeed, just two weeks after his hospitalization for bleeding, he was admitted once again, a fulminating pneumonia sapping the little reserve he had left. Not having suffered enough, he was barely home three days when he returned to the ER, so weak he could not stand even with a walker. His red blood cell count was gravely depleted. His severe anemia required four units of blood and an additional six days of respite on the oncology ward. That provided the tiny bit of energy that allowed him, at least, the dignity of using the toilet without assistance. He'd again required life-saving blood one week ago. Mrs. Lieberman burst into tears when I had called to check on their progress.

"Dear God, I thought I was going to lose him for sure. He was so weak it took me an hour to get him from the house to the car. His lips were blue, and he couldn't breathe. His blood pressure was 86/50 and his heart raced at 120 beats per minute. I should have called an ambulance, but he wouldn't let me. I thought he was going to die."

After she finished, I said quietly, "He was in shock from the low blood cell count."

"I know that now. He had to receive four more units of blood. Dear Lord, how much longer can this go on?"

His brave wife felt so helpless. Thankfully, a close friend was a nurse, and Sheila Lieberman leaned on her like a helpless infant. Not only were they forced to deal with the complications of his disease, but they were also feeling the pinch of a decreased income.

Now, to see them in this place... I walked over and gave each of them a hug.

"It's almost over," Sheila Lieberman said bravely. "We're nearing the end of chemotherapy. The oncologist will keep a very close eye on his blood counts the next couple of weeks and admit him if there's even a hint of what we went through last week."

"Congratulations on being near the end of chemotherapy! It's been a very long haul for both of you. Stan, are you scheduled for any radiation treatments?"

"It hasn't been decided yet. But I had an MRI yesterday, and everything looks clear. No more signs of tumor."

"That's absolutely wonderful. I hope it's downhill from here."

I gave them more hugs before turning away. I'd brought a couple of boxes of chocolate for the oncology nurses. In my experience, nurses never turned down chocolate. At least, I never had. Patty seemed happy to see me and wished me well. I knew I would be returning to the office every three months for the next year before graduating to six-month visits with Dr. Sitarik. I hadn't asked how long the six-month visits would continue, because I wanted to savor each day and didn't want to look too far into the future. I was more than ready to move forward. As Dr. Sitarik said, "What could possibly go wrong now?"

Chapter 32 – Epilogue - March 12th, 2001

Without batting an eye, Bill generously paid for a trip to New York City so I could enjoy Gabriel Byrne's return to the stage in *A Moon for the Misbegotten*. I met yer man on March 7, 2000, after his first performance at the Walter Kerr Theatre. During the play, he poured out his heart for the audience. He *was* James Tyrone, Jr., and Eugene O'Neill would have been proud.

After each show, he, along with the stupendous Cherry Jones and fabulous Roy Dotrice, came out to meet fans and sign autographs. Over the course of four evenings, Mr. Byrne graciously signed several pictures and the new copy of *Pictures in My Head* I'd brought; the copy I'd clung to and read during each chemotherapy session had suffered serious weathering from my sweaty palms and frequent page turning.

I tried out a few Irish phrases in a note I sent backstage and even found myself uttering a couple during the brief chats I had with him while he signed pictures. Since my Irish was rudimentary, I resorted to using a few catchy phrases I'd read in books—sure not to fool anyone who spoke Irish as well as Gabriel Byrne.

"*Dia duit*, Mr. Byrne," I said, so nervously I mispronounced the Irish phrase for hello. Yer man could have corrected me or given me a condescending look for my error, but he didn't. He paused for a second, smiled at me, and said "*Dia duit*, Pamalla," pronouncing the greeting exactly as I had. It was a magnanimous gesture, characteristic, I believe, of his kind and generous spirit.

Instead of returning to Colorado after savoring *Moon* for the final time, I headed to South Carolina to see my dad. Right before the Friday evening performance of *Moon*, my sister Linda had called and told me dad was in the hospital. He'd been suffering chest pain again and needed a four-vessel heart bypass.

When I called my boss, Ruth, in tears, to tell her I needed to detour to South Carolina, she reassuringly said, "Take whatever time you need. Don't worry about a thing." Ruth is the clinic manager everyone dreams of being blessed with. I ended up spending two weeks in South Carolina, because somehow having the family nurse practitioner stay with Dad assured him that leaving the hospital would be okay. I'd be there if anything happened.

Dad did just fine; I'm not sure whether my being there helped him or me more.

I finally returned home to Bill and my new-old car. He'd found my dream car via the Internet during my trials with chemotherapy, and it arrived from Ohio just as my radiation treatments ended—a 1978 Mercedes 450 SL. It's a classic, just like the broad who drives it. Every time I climb behind the wheel of my little Mercedes, I reflect on my good fortune in marrying a man who, since my cancer diagnosis, believes his primary job in life is to make me happy. Hopefully, no one will enlighten him.

Within a few months of completing my miserable chemo treatments and receiving my car, I met an amazing woman, and because of her, many new friends. The woman was Anne Marie Kennedy, an Irishwoman from County Galway with an indefatigable spirit and boundless energy. She absolutely thrived on the excitement she generated in others. Everyone, including me, flourished under her banners of enthusiasm and joy. We met while she was managing a brewery in Louisville. Not busy enough, she was signing up people for an Irish language class. I was determined to get on the list and I did.

The fateful Friday afternoon we met, she, astutely aware I lacked the telltale accent of a native Irishwoman, asked about my interest in Ireland. Despite the busy lunch hour, we spent more than half an hour talking, starting with Gabriel Byrne ("Sure he's a lovely person."), and ending up with a movie we both adore, *Waking Ned Devine* ("We're just after introducing a new beer here in the brewery called Tullymore in honor of that movie."). We've been great friends ever since—the "great" part might all be in my mind, but she puts up with me on a regular basis.

In spite of all she does, she never forgets a birthday or the anniversary of one of her friends. Last month, I was quietly seated in Fadó Irish Pub, waiting for *The Three Irish Chancers'* second set—the *Chancers* are my favorite Irish pub group—when I heard, "Happy Birthday to you…" In came Anne Marie, an Irish hurling stick hoisted above her head, accompanied by dear friends and more gifts. *The Three Irish Chancers*: James Kennedy (Anne Marie's beloved husband), Jim Abbott, and Michael Littwin signed the hurling stick. Handing me the hurling stick, Anne Marie said seriously, "Before the lads signed it, we mucked around in the dirt with it for a bit to give it an authentic look." James was disappointed she would not allow him to *really* authenticate it by adding a few patches of blood and hair, but she drew the line. And no one with any intelligence messes with an Irishwoman who's drawn the line!

Yesterday, I spent ten hours in Anne Marie's company, volunteering at the Mile High Hooley, which featured *bia*, *ól*, and *craic* (food, drink, and Irish fun). Fadó ran out of food and beer, because there were so many people, and much of that was due to Anne Marie's enthusiasm and magnetic personality.

Anne Marie manages two fabulous local Irish groups: *Siúcra* and *The Three Irish Chancers*. *Siúcra* bill themselves as purveyors of quality Irish music, and Shannon and Matthew Heaton and Beth Leachman are every inch quality musicians. Their CD, *"A Place I Know,"* is fabulous. Not wanting to run out, I believe I have fifteen copies.

I took a few tin whistle lessons from Shannon and *bodhrán* (Irish drum) lessons from Matthew. I've heard it said that those who have no musical talent play the *bodhrán*—you disagree, don't you, James Kennedy (*bodhrán* player extraordinaire for *The Three Irish Chancers*)? I'm laughing here, because James is such a humble man, he'd probably blush at the thought of my putting that in print.

The Three Irish Chancers are the rowdiest, happiest, most fun-loving bunch of beer-guzzling singers of traditional pub songs this side of the Emerald Isle. James Kennedy hails from County Galway; Jim Abbott is from County Antrim; and Michael Littwin comes from "the far, far west of Ireland: County Chicago". The fact that a Protestant from the North of Ireland and a Catholic from the South of Ireland are such good friends says much about the hope they generate that all Irish men and women will find joy in one another, regardless of religion or politics. The *Chancers'* first CD was launched at the hooley, and I'm thrilled Bill and I had a tiny part in that undertaking.

I write daily, now that I've made peace with my computer. Actually, Bill bought me a new laptop, so making peace with it merely involved bestowing a Sign of the Cross over it. It was either that or invite an exorcist to deal with the demon who had possessed my first laptop. Bill wasn't convinced the Catholic Church would go for an exorcism of twentieth century hardware, so he splurged on the new equipment. I've finished a novel, and although it hasn't been sold, a publisher is considering it. A couple of dozen people have read it, and they love it. And no, they aren't all friends I've bribed. I'm hopeful.

I wrote the novel, *The Parting Glass*—mentioned here in case you love my droll sense of humor and it gets published before this book does—in between the first vision of this book and the finished version. Interestingly, at least to me, I first wrote *Why Not Me?* as a novel. Looking back, I imagine I was too close to the subject of cancer to feel comfortable saying "I". At least, that's my excuse for not getting it right the first time. There was little of myself in that first book; the facts were there, but I kept my emotions to myself. Since I wrote it while I was undergoing therapy, I worried that spilling my emotions on manuscript pages would result in my inability to control frequent tears and episodes of depression. There was no humor in the book, either. There is nothing humorous about breast cancer, but I live my life surrounded by laughter, and I wanted to share that in the book. This is a much closer version of myself, and I like it more.

In September of 2000, Bill and I spent two glorious weeks in Ireland. We barely dented the surface of what I wanted to see, but I had several missions, as Bill called them, and I accomplished all but one. I could write an entire book about the fabulous places we visited and the friends we made, and maybe I will. I'll be returning twice this year, followed by a trip to Germany to visit long-lost relatives in 2002. There's no moss growing on this breast cancer survivor, unless there's a bit attached to the padded chair where I type my stories.

After my first battle, I often wondered if I would seek treatment for another malignant breast lump or figure once around was enough and go the experimental/cleansing diet route. In June of 2000, I discovered another lump, and the tears and panic I experienced until I was cleared by mammogram and ultrasound made it apparent to me I'm not ready to leave this life without a fight. For those around me, I hope I will experience death in a dignified manner, but mentally, God will have to drag me kicking and screaming to my eternal reward.

I take my tamoxifen daily like the good patient I try to be and suffer hot flashes with only a bit of disgruntlement, putting on and ripping off sweaters and shirts many times in the course of a day. Bill thinks it's cute when he wakes up during the night to see my side of the quilt wadded in the center of the bed, only to have me replace it, shivering, a couple of minutes later. Cute! There's nothing cute about feeling like I'm roasting on a spit one minute and sitting naked at the North Pole the next. My man has an odd idea of what constitutes cute. In his defense, however, at least his idea of cute isn't chasing some twenty-something blonde wearing a skirt that barely covers the essentials and a blouse that is stretched taut against saline-enhanced boobs.

Other than a busted internal thermostat and a horrible fixation on food, which I blame on the tamoxifen, but is more likely attributable to my pathetic refusal to count calories, I have had few side effects from the medication and hope it prevents further cancer. My emotional roller coaster finally leveled out, although some might say I'm as big a pain in the ass as I ever was. However, my dives into the cesspool of despair are rare now. When I'm a bit down, Gloria Bachelder says something helpful like, "Do you really think you're above hormones, Pam?"

I dutifully visit Dr. Sitarik as directed, and I've graduated to check-ups every six months—knock on wood. He pronounces me in good health after poking, prodding, and reviewing lab work. Of course, he doesn't say: "You're clear of cancer", and I know his optimistic remarks don't mean there isn't a little tumor or two lurking around in my body somewhere, but I don't have the time to think about little beasties' invasions. At least visits to his office ensure me I've still got a while. I happened to peek at my chart and noticed this comment for 6/00: "The patient is doing well without obvious evidence of recurrent disease approximately one year after completion of chemotherapy." It's coming up on two years! Yes!

My short-term memory lags are the most emotionally painful. I call them lags, because I eventually recall whatever I need—even if it takes a thesaurus, dictionary, and act of God. But between the elusive beginning and crystallizing endpoint, I sometimes feel like a *fecking eejit*, as James Kennedy might say. When I'm trying to remember a name, a phrase, or where I laid the only pen in the house that hasn't evaporated into thin air, I pace, mumble, talk to the dogs, and try everything short of banging my head against the wall to recall the slippery piece of data. I've resorted to carrying a small notebook in which I jot down timely reminders and phrases I want to slip into some book passage—something that will make me sound infinitely more intelligent than I feel some days. Occasionally, I review what has been written and think, "That sounds really good!" I note it's my handwriting but sometimes can't recall writing it.

Bill kids me when I complain about my poor brain. "You used to be brilliant, Pam," he says. "Now you're functioning at the same level as the rest of us poor, average bastards." He's good at cheering me up.

However, if my cancer remains in remission, even for a few years, I'll be grateful. I suspect I'll get some mileage out of my forgetfulness as I get older. I will be much more likely to elicit sympathy from my grandchildren for missing a school awards' assembly by blaming chemo- therapy rather than owning up to the reality of brain farts, cerebral clutter, or good old-fashioned senility.

Speaking of cancer, I lost Holly to osteosarcoma a month after I completed cancer treatments myself, and my beloved Heidi is suffering the final stages of lymphoma. With three of us having cancer within two years, I sometimes raise my face to heaven and ask, "Okay, whom did I piss off?" Of course, I'm glad that Bill and the children have been spared any serious illness, but I've held three dear dogs as they were put to sleep in the last seventeen years, and it never gets any easier, believe me. I suspect that putting Heidi down will be the most difficult.

The great thing about dogs is they don't know they have cancer and are supposed to act sick. Heidi still enjoys her walks and chases her ball, although her stamina is poor. However, when she collapses on the floor, pooped, she's always sporting a big smile. As long as she's happy, I'll keep her as comfortable as possible. Chemo didn't help her much; she came out of remission within three months. I spend as much free time with her as possible, but occasionally, I need a few hours of mind-numbing, blissful entertainment to comfort me.

I usually fill those hours hollering, singing, stamping my feet, pounding the table, and whistling at *The Three Irish Chancers* during their gigs around the area. Bill, a quiet man, says little other than, "You're certainly enthusiastic, Pam," but I imagine I mortify him. I try not to shout in his ear, but it's his fault if he sits downwind from me. The *Chancers* have promised they'll let me travel with them when they embark on their first Irish tour, but I don't know if they really want my loud-mouthed American enthusiasm embarrassing them in the pubs over there. The lads will probably try to sneak out of the States quietly, without telling me, but I'll be watching the airport. I sometimes wonder if the Irish people will appreciate my T-shirt sporting a picture of *The Three Irish Chancers* on the front and *#1 Groupie* on the back. Hopefully, Irish men and women will have had a few pints in them before our arrival and will chalk me up as a "*fecking Yank*" and leave it at that. I can behave when required, but it takes a lot of effort, and I can't sustain it for long.

Occasionally, Bill and I enjoy a movie when the *Chancers* aren't playing. A few months ago, we took in a comedy at a local movie theater. For the life of me, I can't remember the film, because what happened, before the movie started, spoiled my day. I was in a mindset to have a great time and laugh *me arse* off. However, one of the first ads displayed a request for breast cancer research funds. In huge letters, the audience was reminded that *40,000 women will die of breast cancer this year!* I wanted to scream, "Tell me how many of us are going to live!" I didn't enjoy the movie, and I haven't been back to that theater since.

Yes, we must always, always remember those who have died, some of whom subjected themselves to painful research to benefit those of us who have lived. I mourn those who succumb to this disease. But I want the world to remember that many, many more of us are alive today because of breast cancer research, and the prognosis for a long and healthy life improves each year. I ask people to support breast cancer research, because one day it will guarantee a longer life for a loved one. I ask friends to send checks for breast cancer research to the local American Cancer Society or to one of the many other outstanding foundations supporting breast cancer survivors like the Susan G. Komen Foundation. Buy a breast cancer stamp. Hug a breast cancer survivor—female or male.

Krystal Reider and members of her family participated in last year's Susan G. Komen walk for breast cancer research. Allowed to honor an individual who suffered breast cancer by displaying the name on a shirt, Krystal wore my name. It made me quite proud to be remembered in that way. Krystal will make a fabulous nurse.

More than once, I've asked friends or relatives of a woman with cancer to consider holding a turban party for her. I was thrilled to see that very suggestion in *Dear Abby* a couple of weeks ago. The American Cancer Society has a lovely catalogue called *"TLC"* that's full of hats, turbans, scarves, and wigs to help women with cancer feel beautiful again. Invariably, laughter is shared, and I most assuredly believe sharing heartfelt laughter is essential for recovery.

Many branches of the American Cancer Society also provide free make-up and wig sessions, which are hosted by local experts who selflessly volunteer their time, like my friend Kari, my hairdresser. How uplifting for women (or liberated men) in need of a self-esteem boost!

Since I haven't come up with additional stalling techniques, I'm back at work full-time. My patients seem happy about it, and I am devoted to them, although I must admit writing fulfills a powerful inner need. However, those pesky bills don't pay themselves, and I'm grateful to work at a job I love.

The Family Medical Center staff moved into a fabulous new building on February 5th of this year. Yes! It has eighteen exam rooms (three of which are mine), a huge nurse's station, two procedure rooms, a beautiful waiting room, and a large kitchen. The wallpaper is intact and the carpet is beautiful. So far, no one's puked or had diarrhea on the new furniture—that will come in time, I'm sure.

All the providers have their own offices—even me. Jim Richard is right next door, however, if I need to share a joke or run some ethical question by him. Sharon Pittenger and Dave Hibbard are down the hall. Gloria Bachelder is two doors down, and her son Nicholas occasionally visits. I hadn't seen him for a couple of months, because I had a bit of surgery the end of December; when I returned to work, many patients worried there'd been an exacerbation of my cancer, and their expressions of concern touched me deeply.

Last week, Gloria picked up Nicholas from daycare before returning to the office to complete charts. She assured him I'd still be at work, but she forgot to mention that to me. Having stayed until eight-thirty p.m. on Tuesday, I'd scooted out Wednesday evening at five-thirty. Nicholas arrived, ran to my office, and asked, "Where's Miss Pam?" When told I'd already left, he demanded that Gloria bring him to my house "right now!" We did lunch on Thursday. Lord, I'd forgotten what chasing a four-year-old kid around the playground was like. Maybe I'm not ready for grandkids.

The building that houses our office also boasts an urgent care across the hall. They kindly cater to our needs for stat blood work, X-rays, and ultra-sounds. The patients seem happy. The staff, for the most part, is happy. Of course, we continue to suffer the same aggravating tribulations thanks to a plethora of insurance companies. That probably won't change in my life-time, but nothing's perfect.

I cared for some devastatingly sick patients during my own trials with cancer, and I wrestled with my audacity in believing I had a story worth telling. I kept thinking of Barb and what she might tell me at work: "Don't talk about yourself, Pam; we'll do that after you go home." I am not an extraordinary individual, but I am rich beyond measure thanks to the many lives I've been privileged to touch. I am perpetually grateful for the many friends who bring happiness and humor to my life daily. I have patients who, no matter how sick, never cross my exam room door without a joke to share. Through the years, they have come to know that laughter is as vitally important to my emotional and physical well being as breathing.

There were many times during 1999 that I found little to laugh about. Looking back, joy surrounded me in the form of family and friends, but I was too self-absorbed to appreciate their efforts until later. I still laugh when people tell me how much they admired my strength during that year— it would not have been the way I characterized myself. If I showed any strength at all, it came from those around me, my rocks of fortitude, who shared affection, time, and beliefs that I would get better.

I am, of course, most grateful to my devoted family. Bill and I are closer than we ever have been, and that is good considering our darling children are all preparing to leave the nest. They make my heart soar whenever I think of them. No mother could be prouder of her children's many accomplishments.

I wish to emphasize that delight and joy can return, especially if nurtured and encouraged by friends. But it takes time and patience. It took two years to finish this book, because I could not offer hope when I struggled to find hope for myself. Of course, the degree to which enjoyment of life returns depends on the prognosis one is given, and some aren't as lucky as I have been. If I can offer one personal wish, it is this: please check for early signs of breast and testicular cancer. Please encourage wives, girlfriends, and daughters to get yearly Paps. Pay attention to your body's warning signs. The earlier cancer is detected and treatment undertaken, the better the prognosis for a long and happy future.

Life now is grand—almost perfect, just the way it is. Of course, that doesn't mean I won't try changing things, because I'd hate to become complacent. I treasure my life, my family, and my friends, and I love the direction my life's road has taken. Not bad for a young woman from North Carolina who couldn't decide what to do with her life a short quarter of a century ago. Has it really been that long?

Thoughts of breast cancer never completely leave anyone who has been through what I have—and there are many of us. But I don't think about it all the time. I have the choice of either wrapping myself in a cocoon, isolated from the world, or seizing whatever time I have left and running with it. I have chosen the latter. I hope I have many more years to contribute something meaningful to this world. However, if the time I have left on earth proves to be short, I will have no regrets. I have experienced an amazing amount of love and couldn't ask for more. Okay, I could ask, but I'm probably not going to get it. *Go raibh maith agat!* (Thank-you!)

P.S. In case you're wondering, "Stan Lieberman" had an amazing recovery. The man is a walking miracle, and all who love him are very grateful.

ISBN 155369113-X